What People Are Saying About *The Living Gluten-Free Answer Book* . . .

"Honest, clear, accessible, thoughtful, insightful, and loaded w͏̶   ͏̶eful information, *The Living Gluten Free Answer Book* is by far the ͏̶   seen for
gluten-free beginners, and the people who love and s͏̶   ͏̶wland
brings a tremendously fresh approach to the glut͏̶   ͏̶good
food, an upbeat and positive style, and a s͏̶   ͏̶nity for
those new to the gluten free lifestyle. A͏̶   ͏̶vo!"
Marc David—Nutritional Psychologist, a͏̶   *͏̶ a Diet: Eating for*
Pleasure, Energy and Weight Loss a͏̶   *͏̶isdom: A Mind-Body*
A͏̶   *͏̶o Nutrition and Well Being*

"Everything you ever wanted to know about living gluten-free is right here in this
conveniently-organized, easy-to-read book."
Carol Fenster, PhD, author of *Gluten-Free Quick & Easy* and the forthcoming
1000 Gluten-Free Recipes

"There's a wealth of new information about living well without gluten in this
meticulously-researched guide. It's an encyclopedia for celiacs!"
Jacqueline Mallorca, author of *The Wheat-Free Cook, Gluten-Free*
Recipes for Everyone

"*The Living Gluten-Free Answer Book* will educate food service professionals (from the
baker, cook, and the table server) in realizing that the gluten-free lifestyle is not a fad,
nor a passing moment developed by the world wide web. Anyone mystified about
celiac disease or gluten-intolerance has a great road map to guide them in their quest
to live, eat, and survive without gluten."
Richard J. Coppedge Jr., CMB, Professor in Baking and Pastry,
The Culinary Institute of America, Hyde Park, New York

"As a chef, I am always looking for new experiences, interesting ingredients and unique
preparations. My adventure with gluten-free cooking started with meeting Suzanne
Bowland. Her wealth of knowledge helped me open up the creative flood gates with
new ingredients such as amaranth flour, tapioca flour and Expandex. *The Living Gluten-*
Free Answer Book is not just for people that have gluten intolerance but for all foodies
that are interested in learning about fresh new ingredients and methods of preparation."
Elise Wiggins, Executive Chef, Panzano Restaurant, Denver, Colorado

"*The Living Gluten-Free Answer Book* is an amazing compendium of detailed answers and how-tos for the activities of daily gluten-free living: how to start, how to eat, how to eat out, and how to take control of your life if you need or want to be gluten-free."

John La Puma, MD, Founder, www.glutenfreequiz.com and co-author, *The RealAge Diet* and *Cooking the RealAge Way*

"If you've recently been diagnosed with celiac disease or even merely suspect that you may be gluten-intolerant, you've got a long list of urgent questions. Consider them asked and answered. Suzanne Bowland has amassed a wealth of knowledge in nearly seven years of living gluten-free and shares it in *The Living Gluten-Free Answer Book*. The book will not only spare the newly diagnosed from engaging in weeks, months, or even years of often fruitless fact-finding missions and frustrating experimentation, it may also offer new tips and tricks on every aspect of gluten-free living for people who already know the basics. It's an invaluable guide, both for gluten-intolerant individuals and the healthcare professionals who care for them."

Kate Jackson, Editor, *Today's Diet & Nutrition*

"This is an incredible book for someone newly diagnosed with gluten intolerance or Celiac disease. It is also helpful for someone who has heard of the disease and wants to find out more. This is a one-stop shopping book that provides a wealth of information for those with gluten sensitivity, gluten intolerance and celiac disease."

Renee Zonka, C.E.C., R.D. M.S., Associate Dean, *Kendall College*

THE LIVING GLUTEN-FREE

ANSWERBOOK™

Practical Answers to 275 of Your Most Pressing Questions

SUZANNE BOWLAND

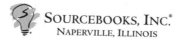

SOURCEBOOKS, INC.®
NAPERVILLE, ILLINOIS

Published by Sourcebooks, Inc.
P.O. Box 4410, Naperville, Illinois 60567-4410
(630) 961-3900
Fax: (630) 961-2168
www.sourcebooks.com

Library of Congress Cataloging-in-Publication Data

Bowland, Suzanne.
  The living gluten-free answer book : answers to 275 of your most pressing questions / by Suzanne Bowland.
    p. cm.
  Includes bibliographical references.
  1. Gluten-free diet--Miscellanea. I. Title.

RM237.86.B69 2008
615.8'54--dc22
                          2007038163

Printed and bound in the United States of America.
VP 10 9 8 7 6 5

Acknowledgments

While writing a book can be a solitary adventure for the author, it's a huge undertaking that is rarely completed without the unwavering support and encouragement of loved ones. I would like to thank my husband, Kelly Bowland. Your love, support, enthusiasm, confidence, suggestions, patience, and countless hours of assistance mean the world to me. And when the daily to-do lists seemed insurmountable at times, and there were many, you always said I would do the right thing, the answers were within me, and I would find them—I did. You continue to inspire me with your strength and love. I love you!

And I would also like to thank my father who has always said to me: *You can do anything you set your mind to.* Dad, you're right! And I admire your sense of patience. It is a virtue. And Mom, thank you for all you have done in my life. I am deeply grateful and I love you both.

A very warm thank you to all of the brilliant chefs, cookbook authors, entrepreneurs, and industry experts who never cease to amaze and inspire me in their creative talents, passion, and expertise in the area of gluten-free cooking, baking, and beyond. You are a joy to learn from and I consider myself so fortunate to know so many of you. All of you are proof positive that the gluten-free food movement is a wonderfully delicious experience to be treasured and enjoyed each day of the journey. A special thanks to Richard Coppedge of The Culinary Institute of America, Marc David, Carol Fenster of Savory Palate, Inc., Jacqueline Mallorca, Lorna Sass, Joel and Mary Schaefer of Walt Disney World, Chef Eric Stein of Johnson & Wales University, Lee Tobin of Whole Foods Market Gluten-Free

Bakehouse, Executive Chef Elise Wiggins of Panzano, and Renee Zonka of Kendall College. You bring new meaning to *Bon Appétit*, gluten-free style.

And a world of gratitude to Dennis Gilliam of Bob's Red Mill Natural Foods who believed in the First Annual Gluten-Free Culinary Summit when I presented the opportunity in 2006. Although not readily apparent, Dennis, you had a part in helping this book become a reality. Had it not been for the First Annual Gluten-Free Culinary Summit that was fueled by the objective to take the gluten-free food movement to the next level of national awareness via the culinary arts, which then lead to the Art & Science of Gluten-Free Gastronomy Lecture Series, I may not have had the opportunity to thank the next individual to whom I'm very grateful.

A heartfelt thank you to my literary agent, Jacky Sach, who presented me with an opportunity to write about my life's passion. I am so appreciative to you for asking me if I would be interested. And to think I may have missed your first email asking about the book had I not checked my spam filter regularly! It brings to mind that there must have been an element of fate at work. The rest, of course, is history. Thank you!

Finally, I would like to thank my publisher, Sourcebooks, Inc., for asking me to take the title of this book you had in mind and run with it. I admire your vision for bringing this timely topic to the marketplace via the question and answer format. It's been a true calling for me. But writing the manuscript is just the beginning. I would like to give a huge thank you to the incredible team of editors at Sourcebooks, Inc.: Shana Drehs, Erin Nevius, and Dojna Shearer. Erin, a special thanks to you for your thoughtful edits, queries, and special touches in the first review. I couldn't have asked for a better team to make this book a reality. Thank you.

Dedication

To the love of my life, best friend, and husband,
Kelly Bowland

My loving parents

And to those who live and are yet to live the gluten-free lifestyle

Contents

Introduction

In March 2001, I began to live life.

For most of my life I suffered from an array of mysterious, chronic symptoms that would never dissipate despite my best efforts, from going to doctors to trying to relieve symptoms on my own. I was chronically fatigued, but forced myself to exercise daily until exhaustion as a way to feel better, and still the symptoms persisted. Eating a healthy, all-natural diet was a way of life for me, but the symptoms lingered. I never felt my best. Doctors would guess at what caused the symptoms and would inconclusively provide a different diagnosis each time, ranging from lactose intolerance and ulcers to anxiety and depression. I saw more doctors than I care to count. They remained baffled and I began to regard feeling bad as a way of life—for me anyway. It was sad.

Then one day, everything changed. I decided to embark upon an "elimination diet" for the sole purpose of losing a couple of pounds to feel better in my clothes—I thought shedding some weight could at least curb the persistent bloat and stomach distress. I ended up losing much more than a couple pounds. I lost a way of life that had put a damper on my physical well-being and outlook on life and instead gained a whole new way of living, symptom-free.

I eliminated dense carbohydrate foods from my diet, including those made with flour or starch. Along with rice, corn, and potatoes, I also eliminated anything with flour for about two weeks. I didn't recognize at that time that I was eliminating wheat and gluten. I fought the urge to feast on bread, pasta, cereal, crackers, and all sweet and savory freshly baked and processed foods. It was a difficult adjustment indeed, but I believed that a strict diet of meat, fish, eggs, nuts, fruits, and vegetables would get rid of those pounds and might even make me feel better. I have always been mindful of nutritious eating and had read in many publications that eating a non-processed diet was a particularly healthy approach, and I figured now was the time to adopt it, as nothing else had helped.

Soon, I discovered this diet was more than a quick trick to lose a couple pounds. It was a miracle. But the true discovery came after a little bump in the road to recovery.

After eating this self-prescribed diet for several days, I began to feel great. Marvelous would be a better adjective! But I still had no idea that the elimination of wheat and gluten was the secret, and I decided it was time to celebrate. After approximately a couple weeks, I had shed a few pounds, the bloat was gone, the brain fog had lifted, my mood was blissful, and the gastrointestinal stress I took as being a natural way of life for me had *finally* disappeared. I felt genuinely energetic, not lethargic. Happy days were here! My diet had worked.

To reward myself, I soon thereafter indulged in a food I had been missing: a bowl of my favorite cereal. But then the unimaginable happened. Virtually moments later, I had to lie down—my cramping and other symptoms returned with a vengeance, and my blissful mood plummeted. I was dumbfounded, but mostly disappointed— very disappointed. A couple weeks of feeling physically wonderful were quickly erased by one bowl of cereal.

While miserably battling my old symptoms and contemplating what might have happened, a little light came on inside my head. It didn't take long for me to put two and two together, and I guessed at the common denominator in this scenario—it had to be wheat! I promptly headed to my computer to Google the term "wheat allergy." Pages and pages of information on the topic unfolded before me. As I read on, I was thrilled to learn about wheat/gluten-intolerance and celiac disease; it finally provided me with the answers I had been seeking for so many years. As I read through the symptoms and personal stories of wheat/gluten-intolerance, I related. That's me! That's how I feel! Mystery solved.

I was like a sponge for information on the topic, and I discovered a small selection of foods I could eat and where to buy them in my city and on the Internet. The quest for information continued and in the meantime, I vowed never to eat or drink anything that contained gluten again. The symptoms of the infamous "cereal celebration" soon dissipated and I began living symptom free again. I am now approaching seven years of living gloriously gluten, and symptom, free.

When I discovered my intolerance to gluten in March 2001, my life entered a new phase that can be described as nothing less than a true renaissance—an evolution in well-being. With the disappearance of my symptoms, I could actually feel my body heal and delight in the glory of being happy and human without having to succumb to physical distress.

While I could go on and on about how the gluten-free life has been my saving grace and how it has improved and enhanced my life in countless ways, I urge anyone who experienced or currently experiences just one of the chronic symptoms associated with gluten-intolerance or celiac disease (see page 6 for a list of symptoms) to take action now. Visit your doctor and request a blood test to determine if you are intolerant to gluten and take the next steps to a diagnosis and following a gluten-free diet. You can't afford to wait.

For those of you who pick up this book to learn more about the gluten-free lifestyle that you are now pursuing, I wrote the contents with you in mind. I know you have many questions—years ago I had the same questions. I want to provide you with the information, tips, tools, and strategies you'll need as you embark upon a gluten-free journey, for whatever reason you're beginning to follow the diet. You don't have to learn the ropes, one by one, over the course of several years like I did. These answers will save you a considerable amount of time and guesswork. The pages within can serve as your blueprint for making one of the most poignant transitions in your life— one that can be the start of a personal evolution in health and well-being like nothing you've experienced before, and one that millions are experiencing right now and millions more are yet to discover and relish. You hold the keys, and I invite you to enjoy the deliciously abundant journey.

Best wishes to you in living gluten-free!

Suzanne Bowland
Denver, Colorado

Chapter 1

GLUTEN-INTOLERANCE: WHAT IS IT?

- What is gluten-intolerance and celiac disease?
- Can you be gluten-intolerant but not celiac?
- Then what is gluten sensitivity?
- What is dermatitis herpetiformis?
- Are gluten-intolerance and celiac disease hereditary?
- What are the symptoms of gluten-intolerance?
- What should you do if you think you are gluten-intolerant?
- Can you have celiac disease and not know it?
- If celiac disease remains undiagnosed, what can happen?
- Why are gluten-intolerance and celiac disease underdiagnosed?
- What causes gluten-intolerance or celiac disease?
- Can you develop celiac disease later in life?
- Can you prevent celiac disease from developing if you know you are genetically predisposed?
- Is there a cure for celiac disease?
- Is there a cure for gluten-intolerance?
- Can you "outgrow" gluten-intolerance or celiac disease?
- Are certain nationalities more predisposed to gluten-intolerance than others?
- Are females more at risk than males for being gluten-intolerant or developing celiac disease?
- How many people in the United States have celiac disease?
- How many people in the United States have nonceliac gluten-intolerance?
- What are the diagnostic tests for celiac disease?
- What is the "gluten challenge"?
- What is genetic testing for celiac disease?
- Should you consider genetic testing for celiac disease?
- Is genetic testing for celiac disease covered under health insurance?
- How long does it take to heal after being on the gluten-free diet?

- What other conditions may benefit from the gluten-free diet?
- Does gluten affect the brain?
- What is the difference between a food allergy and a food intolerance?
- Who discovered that wheat was associated with celiac disease?

What is gluten-intolerance and celiac disease?

Defining gluten-intolerance and celiac disease begins with under-standing one basic human function: digestion. A miraculous process of design, the process of digestion takes the foods and beverages we consume, breaks them down, extracts the nutrients, and makes them transportable to nourish our bodies. But like any other process of the human body, digestion can malfunction.

Celiac disease is an autoimmune digestive disorder that causes an inability to digest a specific protein known as *gluten*. Gluten is found in the cereal grain families of wheat, barley, and rye. This inability to process is due mostly to a fragment of gluten known as *gliadin* and begins in the small intestine, the place responsible for much of the digestive and absorption process of foods. Celiac disease is consid-ered to be full-blown gluten-intolerance.

The body is naturally designed to defend itself from foreign or "non-self" invaders to keep healthy. But an autoimmune disease is a condition where the body is tricked into attacking itself, thinking that protein and tissues of the body are "anti-self." In the case of celiac disease, the small intestinal wall lined with villi becomes the victim of the body's self-attack and is visibly damaged.

To illustrate, envision a healthy small intestinal wall lined with little, protruding, fingerlike hairs known as villi. Healthy villi act as the body's welcoming committee for food, granting the entry of necessary nutrients to the rest of the body for survival. But for a body that views gluten as an "anti-self" or foreign substance, the body, or specifically the intestinal wall, turns against itself. The villi respond by refusing entry of gluten through the small intestine. This continual mode of attack on gluten, each time it's consumed, causes inflammation of the villi. With continued consumption of gluten, the villi "flatten," making the surface area of the small intestinal wall abnormally smooth and no longer able to properly digest and absorb all of the valuable nutrients from food as it was designed to do. As a result, the body suffers from a state of malabsorption, and it can experience a multi-faceted range of physically uncomfortable symptoms and long-term complications. This state of intestinal distress is known as celiac disease.

Can you be gluten-intolerant and not celiac?

Yes. While celiac disease is gluten-intolerance to the fullest extent, gluten-intolerance is not necessarily celiac disease. Only a small portion of those who are gluten-intolerant have celiac disease. To accurately define and understand your individual relationship with gluten, it's important to grasp the important distinction between celiac disease, gluten-intolerance, and gluten-sensitivity because they are three different, though similar, conditions.

Celiac Disease

If you have celiac disease, you are gluten-intolerant. Celiac disease is full-blown gluten-intolerance that usually manifests in physical damage of the small intestine (i.e., flattened villi). You can actually *see* celiac disease through a biopsy of the small intestine, which is typically considered to be the ultimate diagnosis for the disease. The intestinal wall appears smooth and lacks the bumpy, fingerlike protrusions known as healthy villi.

Gluten-Intolerance

On the other hand, you can be gluten-intolerant—and therefore gluten-sensitive—but not have celiac disease. While *nonceliac gluten-*

intolerance produces antibodies to gluten and results in many of the same physical symptoms and complications associated with celiac disease, it does not result in physical damage of the small intestinal villi. You can accurately label yourself as gluten-intolerant if you experience uncomfortable symptoms as a result of consuming gluten, and if your symptoms disappear when gluten is removed permanently from your diet. Nonceliac gluten-intolerance symptoms are no less painful or important to treat than celiac disease; your villi are simply not flattened (damaged) as a result of your nonceliac gluten-intolerance.

Then what is gluten sensitivity?

Gluten sensitivity is often used as an umbrella term for anyone who reacts negatively to gluten, including those with celiac disease. But gluten-sensitivity is the "soft" version, compared to the "hard" versions of celiac disease and gluten-intolerance. You can be sensitive to gluten, but not necessarily be gluten-intolerant. Unlike celiac disease and gluten-intolerance, with gluten-sensitivity you can experience fleeting gastrointestinal discomfort or other annoying symptoms, but there is no *dramatic* physical change when gluten is either consumed or removed from the diet. Dramatic is the operative word. Gluten-sensitivity may encourage you to eat less gluten in your diet to feel better, but your symptoms are not as full-blown as the symptoms associated with celiac disease and gluten-intolerance. With gluten-sensitivity, you may choose not to eliminate gluten entirely from your diet and merely accept the occasional discomfort. Gluten-sensitivity may not medically require the removal of gluten from the diet, whereas celiac disease and gluten-intolerance do.

What is dermatitis herpetiformis?

If you are diagnosed with dermatitis herpetiformis, you have a form of celiac disease, but your small intestine *may not* receive the damage. Where celiac disease damages the small intestine, dermatitis herpetiformis wreaks havoc with the skin. Characterized by a severe skin rash that is extremely itchy, dermatitis herpetiformis is distinguished from other rashes with its own brand of blisters and lesions often produced by the incessant scratching of the sufferer. The rash can occur anywhere on the body, but is most found on extremities like the elbows and knees. The condition is diagnosed through a skin biopsy using a sample from right next to a lesion, but not directly from the lesion itself.

As with celiac disease, dermatitis herpetiformis is an autoimmune disorder that erupts with the ingestion of gluten; even the smallest trace can produce a severe reaction in extremely sensitive individuals. Those with dermatitis herpetiformis are also more prone to bone disease, as well as the same host of autoimmune disorders that individuals with celiac disease can be predisposed to developing. While dermatitis herpetiformis results in extreme skin irritation, it is also possible to experience intestinal wall damage—a two-fold assault on the body.

Are gluten-intolerance and celiac disease hereditary?

Yes. Gluten-intolerance and celiac disease are genetically predisposed autoimmune conditions. According to Prometheus Therapeutics & Diagnostics in San Diego, California, it's estimated that approximately one third or 37 percent of the population in the United States carries the gene for celiac disease; however, current statistics estimate that one in 133 people actually express the gene and develop the disease. As awareness and the diagnosis rate of celiac disease continue to increase, it's realistic to expect that the 133 statistic will decrease with future studies.

Predicting the probability of an individual developing celiac disease when the gene is present is not an exact science—you can have the gene and never develop the disease. Plus, environmental factors are believed to play a role in the manifestation of the disease, and these factors, namely stress-related factors, vary from individual to individual. Thus, there is no specific formula for predicting the probability of acquiring the gene or developing the condition like there is for attempting to predict one's eye color based on the eye color of the parents. If one or both parents carry the gene, whether or not they will pass the gene onto a child is unpredictable. However, relative to the rest of the population, you are more likely than others to carry the gene if it runs in your immediate family. And it's also possible for a child to carry the gene even if the parents do not. Even with identical twins, there is no predictability. If both carry the gene, one can develop the disease while the other escapes it.

Bottom line: While much remains to be studied about the genetic link to celiac disease, it is at least known for certain that the gene must be present before the disease can manifest.

What are the symptoms of gluten-intolerance?

Gluten-intolerance and celiac disease are two chronic conditions still abysmally underdiagnosed—they have an aura of mystery because everyone who is intolerant to gluten reacts differently to it. There is no cookie-cutter diagnosis of symptoms, and the symptoms and complications of gluten-intolerance often mimic those of other conditions.

If you would like to know whether you are gluten-intolerant, the following list will serve as a starting point to help unravel a mystery in your world and possibly steer you in the right direction. This list categorizes the symptoms by looking at the whole body and dividing it into its elemental areas, listing some of the common, chronic symptoms or complications associated with celiac disease and gluten-intolerance in that area of the body. And keep the word "chronic" in mind, as it's an important term. Chronic implies a severe, prolonged, or returning problem, not just a fleeting or rare discomfort that could be attributed to sensitivity, not intolerance. All of the symptoms listed here are some of the chronic symptoms commonly associated with gluten-intolerance and celiac disease.

1. **Abdomen**
    Recurring intestinal problems that can include one or more of the following: diarrhea, constipation, gas, acid reflux, cramping, stomach pain, stomach upset, bloating, problematic stools

2. **Head**
    Headaches, migraines, brain fog

3. **Skin**
    Itchy skin, rashes or blisters, eczema, mouth sores

4. **Circulatory/Blood**
    Anemia, malabsorption

5. **Skeleton and Muscles**
    Osteoporosis, osteopenia, bone/joint pain, muscle cramps, numbness or tingling in arms, hands, feet, dental enamel problems, stunted growth in children

6. **Reproduction**
    Infertility, irregular menstruation, recurrent miscarriage

7. **Spirit/Energy**
    Chronic, unexplained fatigue, weakness, weight loss, irritability

8. **Mental/Neurological**
   Behavioral issues, seizures, depression, psychiatric problems

9. **Autoimmune System**
   Diabetes, thyroid disease, liver disease

10. **Nervous System**
    Fibromyalgia

11. **Cancer**
    Non-Hodgkin's lymphoma; cancer in small intestine

What should you do if you think you are gluten-intolerant?

If you experience one or more of the above "chronic" symptoms or complications and are currently consuming gluten, a doctor's visit to discuss your situation and options for testing, diagnosis, and the gluten-free diet is well worth it. Don't delay.

It's not advised to undertake the gluten-free diet permanently without an accurate diagnosis. However, if you have already eliminated gluten from your diet and have witnessed a dramatic disappearance of uncomfortable symptoms, congratulations—you are on the right track to making a possible connection to gluten-intolerance. However, you should still see your physician to ensure that you accurately solve the mystery.

Can you have celiac disease and not know it?

Yes—you can experience the uncomfortable symptoms associated with gluten-intolerance or celiac disease but not know it's gluten that is causing the discomfort, which is one of the reasons why the disease is so widely underdiagnosed. However, with celiac disease, symptoms can seem invisible or "silent," making diagnosis even more difficult. It's possible to experience no apparent symptoms associated with celiac disease but have a positive intestinal biopsy or positive blood test for the disease. With nearly three million Americans estimated to have celiac disease and 97 percent unaware of it, this is reason alone to consider the importance of being tested. And it can be as simple as asking your doctor to perform the appropriate blood tests while you are on a gluten-based diet. Testing for celiac disease is not standard operating procedure in doctors' offices, and in most cases the tests will need to be requested by patients who want to have them performed. If you know of anyone in your close family who has celiac disease, you should get tested as soon as possible. And if you don't know if a member of your family has the condition or not, it's still wise to consider testing.

A third of the population is estimated to carry the genetic marker for celiac disease and such a significant statistic provides reasonable grounds to make genetic testing for babies routine, along with other tests they take. Early detection of the marker can guide lifestyle choices centered around the gluten-free diet to help prevent the disease from taking hold in the first place.

If celiac disease remains undiagnosed, what can happen?

As with virtually any condition, if it's left to run its course without treatment, severe complications can result; the worst case scenario being death. In the case of gluten-intolerance and celiac disease, a variety of severe, long-term conditions can manifest themselves above and beyond the everyday physical symptoms of the disease.

Celiac disease is a condition that first affects your gut, the core of your being. This is the place where your life is fed, literally. Proper digestion makes absorption of critical nutrients possible, but if the small intestine is not working properly, malabsorption can lead to malnutrition. So, despite consuming a nutritious diet, critical nutrients such as A, B-12, D, E, K, folate, and iron can't enter the bloodstream, but are excreted, contributing to the possibility of causing anemia (iron deficiency), or stunted growth or developmental problems in children.

Conditions such as osteopenia and osteoporosis are also commonly associated with celiac disease—which leads back to the issue of malabsorption. If calcium and vitamin D, two key nutrients for healthy bones, are continually lost through excretion, your bones will not receive the necessary requirements for proper bone density.

Other complications that can develop as a result of untreated gluten-intolerance and celiac disease include autoimmune disorders, cancer, depression, infertility, neurological disorders, and lactose intolerance. And with such an array of conditions such as these, it begs the question: is celiac disease still underdiagnosed? Unfortunately, the answer is yes.

Why are gluten-intolerance and celiac disease underdiagnosed?

The medical community provides a variety of reasons why gluten-intolerance and celiac disease have proven to be severely underdiagnosed "decoy" conditions. Up until recently, celiac disease has been considered a *rare* disease, not affecting the numbers of people it's now known to affect, let alone the number of unsuspected sufferers. When a disease is out of the public eye, it's often out of the mind, and doctors have regularly overlooked celiac disease as being a cause for the patient's symptoms, because they're looking elsewhere for more "common" conditions or denominators. And if the symptoms are latent, the disease can remain a mystery within the individual.

Since everyone with gluten-intolerance has their own signature set of reactions to gluten, it can be a challenge to diagnose, because there are no specific, unwavering symptoms. Plus, there are a variety of other conditions with symptoms similar to those of gluten-intolerance. Gastrointestinal disorders such as lactose intolerance, irritable bowel syndrome (IBS), and Crohn's Disease cause symptoms similar to gluten-intolerance, but are much more commonly diagnosed. Countless scenarios are surfacing of individuals reporting they've been diagnosed with "anything and everything under the sun," except for the condition masquerading in disguise: celiac disease or gluten-intolerance.

While it's not surprising the general population is still largely unaware of gluten-intolerance and celiac disease, it is surprising that the medical community has been slow to build its own uniform level of awareness. And unfortunately, underdiagnosed and misdiagnosed cases still abound.

What causes gluten-intolerance or celiac disease?

The reasons why people are gluten-intolerant or develop celiac disease are not entirely clear, but it is known that gluten is the activator in this genetically predisposed condition. It's also believed there are other environmental *triggers* that can cause the body to reject gluten, but those specific triggers have not been fully studied and are yet to be confirmed. Some experts believe that stress can be an environmental trigger that may shift the body of someone who is genetically predisposed into a state of permanent gluten-intolerance, and thus becomes more prone to developing celiac disease. And while these stress factors are not exactly understood and defined by the medical community, it's speculated that stress resulting from trauma, injury, infection, or even pregnancy could be a factor. Diet is also a topic of speculation. Could an individual's diet shift the body into a state of stress and therefore make the body more susceptible to becoming gluten-intolerant if the gene is present? Conclusive answers are not yet available and much research remains to be done before the causes and environmental triggers of gluten-intolerance and celiac disease are more clearly understood.

Can you develop celiac disease later in life?

If you have the genetic predisposition for celiac disease, you can develop the condition at any age. The range for expressing the disease is widespread, beginning in early childhood and spanning through late adulthood. There is no common denominator for developing the disease with respect to age.

Can you prevent celiac disease from developing if you know you are genetically predisposed?

This question presents a strong case for the importance of genetic screening for the disease at an early age, before gluten is introduced regularly into the diet. It stands to reason that if you are aware of the genetic possibility of the disease from a young age you can prevent it from manifesting by following a gluten-free diet—if the gluten trigger is not present, the disease has no foothold to begin. Consult with your physician on the best course of action if you have the gene, but don't have the disease.

Is there a cure for celiac disease?

Thankfully, there is a cure for the symptoms and intestinal damage or skin irritation associated with celiac disease, but not the condition itself. The only "cure" is the permanent removal of gluten from the diet so that the small intestine can recover and return to normal functioning. Early diagnosis of celiac disease is critical and the gluten-free diet must be adopted immediately to eliminate symptoms and help prevent further complications associated with the disease.

Is there a cure for gluten-intolerance?

Unfortunately, no. Gluten-intolerance is a permanent condition. Once you are gluten-intolerant or celiac, you are always gluten-intolerant or celiac. But the condition is "cured" by strictly following a gluten-free diet; you'll never be free of it, but the symptoms will cease.

Can you "outgrow" gluten-intolerance or celiac disease?

Even though the gluten-free diet will relieve all of the symptoms of gluten-intolerance, this is still a common question with a definitive answer: no. Celiac disease is an autoimmune condition that remains with you for life, which is why it's so important to strictly maintain a gluten-free diet. But to bring a little light to the equation, it's nice to know you can "outgrow" certain aspects of living with the condition.

Optimists and positive thinkers know you get what you focus on, so in the spirit of optimism, you have the following to look forward to over the course of your gluten-free life (some of these you will outgrow quickly, whereas others may take more time and patience):

- You will outgrow your cravings for wheat-based products, such as cookies, muffins, pizza, breads, and so forth. With time, your memory fades and your taste buds grow accustomed to the taste and texture of similar gluten-free baked goods, particularly when you find ones that you love—and you will!
- You will outgrow your novice approach to avoiding gluten as you become a seasoned expert in the art of bypassing the forbidden protein.

- You will outgrow any anger associated with the rigidity of conforming to a relatively restrictive diet. You can fight it kicking and screaming the whole way, but over time, the anger drains your energy, and you will eventually move into the phase of acceptance and enjoyment of what gluten-free living can offer you.
- Last, but not least, you will outgrow the body once damaged by gluten and acquire a newer, healthier, gluten-free body, without the uncomfortable symptoms you once knew and hated. As your body continues to replace cells throughout your life, you can in essence have a new body! So, even though you won't outgrow the intolerance, you can outgrow much of the cellular damage caused by your intolerance to gluten.

Are certain nationalities more predisposed to gluten-intolerance than others?

The United States, Canada, and Europe share similar statistics with respect to the number of individuals estimated to have the disease. Even though it appears as though individuals affected by or are at risk of developing celiac disease are primarily of European descent, there is no definitive research that suggests one specific nationality is at higher risk than another for developing the disease. Research reveals, however, that celiac disease is rare in individuals of African and Asian descent.

Are females more at risk than males for being gluten-intolerant or developing celiac disease?

There is no indication that gender has any bearing on developing the disease. Both men and women who have the gene for celiac disease share the same risk in developing it. However, according to Dr. Peter H.R. Green, M.D., Director of the Celiac Disease Center at Columbia

University and author of *Celiac Disease—A Hidden Epidemic*, current statistics reveal that more women have autoimmune diseases than men do, and that women with celiac disease outnumber men in a ratio as high as three to one.

How many people in the United States have celiac disease?

Only a small portion of those who are gluten-intolerant have celiac disease. As research continues to be conducted on this surprisingly underdiagnosed condition, the number of people affected continues to increase. The latest research suggests that celiac disease affects one in 133 Americans, which translates into approximately 1 percent of the population or 3 million Americans. Shockingly, 97 percent of those estimated to have celiac disease remain undiagnosed.

How many people in the United States have nonceliac gluten-intolerance?

An exact number is yet to be determined, but estimates are being reported in the high millions, or as many as one in seven people, which is considerably larger than the segment affected by celiac disease.

What are the diagnostic tests for celiac disease?

If you suspect you may be gluten-intolerant or have celiac disease, visiting a doctor that specializes in gastroenterology is a good first step. Going on a gluten-free diet is a serious, life-changing event that requires a sound diagnosis of the condition first, and the most accurate diagnosis is obtained with an intestinal biopsy. It's performed via an endoscopy under conscious sedation. However, before undertaking such an invasive measure, a doctor will generally perform blood tests. (Some doctors may choose to do the biopsy first, based on the nature of the symptoms and family history.)

Without getting technical, there are four specific blood tests for celiac disease that provide highly sensitive results and serve as the first road to diagnosis for the disease. All four tests comprise a panel for blood work that look for antibody levels associated with gluten; the results help determine whether or not a biopsy should be the next step to a diagnosis. Some doctors may consider positive results from the blood tests to be a diagnosis.

The test for dermatitis herpetiformis is a skin biopsy, and is performed at the site of the rash after an outbreak. Should this test be positive, the diagnosis for celiac disease is confirmed and the intestinal biopsy is not needed.

Although not a diagnostic test for celiac disease, genetic testing is a viable alternative for helping to rule out which members of the family will not develop celiac disease. Plus, it's an option for those who have been following a gluten-free diet for a while and don't want to take on the "gluten challenge," in order to produce accurate blood test results, but want more concrete evidence as to whether or not they have the genetic marker for the disease.

What is the "gluten challenge?"

It's common for individuals to go on a gluten-free diet on their own without being medically diagnosed with celiac disease or gluten-intolerance, because of the remarkable disappearance of symptoms on the gluten-free diet. However, it's natural to want to be tested for celiac disease so that you know for sure one way or the other. But in order for blood tests and an intestinal biopsy to be as accurate as possible, gluten must be consumed for a period of time prior to and during testing. Dr. Peter Green, in his book *Celiac Disease, A Hidden Epidemic*, discusses the gluten challenge, stating that it typically requires the individual to consume the equivalent of at least four slices of bread a day for one to four months prior to testing. This time frame should be long enough for the indicators of celiac disease (i.e. damage to the small intestinal wall) to become present and render a blood test or biopsy conclusive.

The gluten challenge can be an uncomfortable scenario to contemplate, as well as undergo, for anyone who has concluded for themselves that gluten is the culprit behind their physical malaise. But the gluten-challenge is a necessary evil if you are after a conclusive diagnosis for celiac disease. For some individuals, taking on the gluten challenge may illicit such uncomfortable physical symptoms that a doctor will not recommended it. Or, if someone has been on the gluten-free diet for several years and symptoms no longer exist, taking on the gluten-challenge may be a moot point—you already know you feel better without gluten, so why subject yourself to the test?

While the prospect of knowing for certain whether or not you have celiac disease may encourage you to take on the gluten challenge, the mere thought of the resulting sickness may be enough to make you content in your uncertainty. Just knowing that the gluten-free diet improved your well-being in dramatic ways may be all you need to know, even though the mystery will still linger. It's a hard decision, but one that should be given serious consideration, particularly if you are trying to determine possible associations to the disease in your family.

What is genetic testing for celiac disease?

When an unsolved mystery is afoot, clues are always welcome. But clues are just that—clues. They can produce a viable hunch and help lead you in the direction of finding the answers to solving the mystery, but they are not the answers themselves.

Genetic test results for celiac disease can either be an *answer* or a *clue*. Genetic testing is a *rule out* test for celiac disease: It does not conclusively determine that you have it; if the test is negative, it rules out the possibility that you have or could develop the disease (an answer). But a positive result means only that you may have celiac disease or could develop it. The test is only an indicator for the possibility of the disease by revealing the presence of the gene, but it is not a diagnosis (only a clue). The ultimate answer is a positive diagnosis through an intestinal biopsy. Keep in mind that you could have the genetic marker and still have a negative intestinal biopsy. This could mean that you may have not developed the disease yet, you may never develop it, or it is latent.

According to Prometheus Therapeutics & Diagnostics in San Diego, California, approximately 37 percent of the United States population has the genetic marker for celiac disease. But not all people who carry the marker will develop the disease. And keep in mind that a negative result does not mean that you are not gluten-intolerant or gluten-sensitive.

Should you consider genetic testing for celiac disease?

Possible Scenario #1: Answer Is No.

If you suspect you may have celiac disease, the first logical step is to visit a physician, preferably one who specializes in gastroenterology, and is highly knowledgeable about the condition. It's often advisable to have a panel of blood tests performed first, to indicate whether or not you have a level of antibodies in your blood consistent with celiac disease. If these are positive, further consultation with your physician will be needed to determine if a gluten-free diet should be started, or if a biopsy should be the next step for a thorough diagnosis. In this case, genetic testing would simply be an extra step that would not be helpful in determining a diagnosis.

Possible Scenario #2: Answer Is Yes.

If you have been on the gluten-free diet for more than six months, blood testing for celiac antibodies could yield a false negative result, because you are not currently consuming gluten. And if you choose to not take the gluten challenge (consume gluten for a period of time) in order to produce accurate blood test results, but you *really* want to know if you might have or could possibly develop the disease, genetic testing is a viable option. It won't tell you for sure that you have it or could develop it, but you will definitely know if the disease is *not* a possibility for you. If all symptoms have cleared up on a gluten-free diet and the genetic test is positive, this may provide you with the information you were looking for, even though it's still not a definitive diagnosis.

Possible Scenario #3: Answer Is Maybe.

If you don't have health insurance, but want to know if you have the genetic marker for celiac disease, it will be a costly out-of-pocket expense. It's up to you how much you want to know, and how much you're willing to pay for the clue.

Possible Scenario #4: Yes.

Getting a genetic test done is a good option if you want to be proactive in determining who in the family has a gene for celiac disease, in order that they can consider the possible advantages of following the gluten-free diet for preventative maintenance.

Is genetic testing for celiac disease covered under health insurance?

Check with your provider, but genetic testing for celiac disease is often insured under preventative maintenance.

How long does it take to heal after being on the gluten-free diet?

Just as the range of symptoms varies for each individual who has celiac disease, the time it takes to heal after going on a gluten-free diet will also vary. But there are two aspects of healing on this diet to consider. Perceived healing is different from actual healing. Those who have suffered from mysterious symptoms for most of their life may recognize a dramatic improvement in well-being once they begin to eliminate gluten from their diet. Many report that their recovery happens rather quickly. This perceived feeling of immediate recovery may be real, but naturally the small intestine will take longer to recover. The speed of the healing depends on the damage done, as well as the severity of possible complications that need attention, such as poor bone density or anemia due to the prolonged malabsorption of nutrients. However, since gluten causes inflammation to the small intestine, the removal of gluten will enable the small intestine to recover to normal functioning quickly, often within weeks.

Others will not respond to the diet as quickly. For those who have celiac disease, but who do not necessarily feel ill when ingesting gluten, their sense of perceived healing may not be all that significant even when the small intestine begins to recover. Not feeling the healing can be frustrating and a detriment to remaining vigilant on the diet, because there seem to be no immediate awards. However, it's important to stick with the diet because, even if you don't feel the healing it is taking place.

What other conditions may benefit from a gluten-free diet?

The strict, lifelong commitment to the gluten-free diet is required for those with celiac disease, and it has been found to be highly beneficial for those with gluten-intolerance. But a gluten-free diet is also being recommended for a broad range of other conditions, either as a form of treatment or as part of an overall program. Much research remains to be done to find conclusive evidence, but a growing body of medical research and individual reports suggest that symptoms associated with the following conditions may subside or be managed by adherence to a gluten-free diet:

- Anemia
- Ataxia
- Attention-Deficit/Hyperactivity Disorder (ADHD)
- Autism
- Autoimmune Diseases
- Cognitive disorders
- Diabetes (Type 1 and Type 2)
- Dementia
- Dental Enamel Defects
- Depression
- Down's syndrome
- Eczema
- Epilepsy
- Fibromyalgia
- Hypothyroidism
- Infertility
- Migraines
- Malignancy
- Multiple sclerosis
- Osteoporosis
- Parkinson's disease
- Peripheral neuropathies
- Psoriasis

- Rheumatoid arthritis
- Sinus problems
- Thyroid Disease (autoimmune)

While more and more doctors begin and continue to recommend the gluten-free diet to help manage the symptoms associated with the above conditions, it is possible that individuals could find out they are gluten-intolerant or have celiac disease via the disappearance of other symptoms, and witness a dramatic improvement in well-being. For example, a California woman reported the disappearance of lifelong gastrointestinal symptoms, after being on the gluten-free diet that was recommended by her doctor to help manage her symptoms associated with multiple sclerosis. And a Denver woman stopped having miscarriages and was able to carry a baby to full term after going on the gluten-free diet recommended by her doctor for infertility issues. She later discovered she had celiac disease, as does her son.

Does gluten affect the brain?

This is a fascinating question with many answers waiting to be revealed through studies yet to be conducted, in and outside the context of celiac disease. But individuals with gluten-intolerance or celiac disease who have reported "brain fog" as a symptom, and found that the "cloud" miraculously lifted after going on the gluten-free diet, will swear that gluten affects their brain.

Individual stories abound in which people, celiac and nonceliac gluten-intolerant alike, found one or more of the following scenarios to be true after permanently following the gluten free diet:

1. Improved concentration and focus; clearer thinking
2. Improved mood and outlook on life; depression lifted

3. Improved interest in learning, memory retention, and intellectual faculty
4. Improved energy level
5. Stopped medications previously prescribed for a psychiatric disorder

Though there is no voluminous body of scientifically supported knowledge that endorses these claims, the answers are undeniably intriguing.

There remains much to be explored about the brain-stomach-gluten connection, and gluten-intolerance is bringing much needed attention to this hypothesis. How does gluten affect the brain tissue and the workings of the brain? Or, how can certain functions in the body, such as digestion, affect the brain when they aren't working properly? Clearly, frequent bouts of gluten-produced abdominal pain can surely be a damper on one's outlook on life!

While research is suggestive of definite links between gluten and the brain, much remains sheer speculation. Perhaps we are simply in the midst of an interesting evolution where science and medicine have not yet caught up to the large body of personal, anecdotal experience that claims beyond a reasonable doubt that gluten affects the brain. Many a gluten-free individual will gladly remain gluten-free to keep their minds happy on many different levels, and they won't wait for the science to prove them correct.

What is the difference between a food allergy and a food intolerance?

It's common to find the words allergy and intolerance used interchangeably—as well as inaccurately—in verbal and written exchanges, but it's important to understand that they mean two different things.

Lets first look at it metaphorically. To understand a *food allergy* via metaphor, envision your body as a castle with a moat and high stone walls that fortify the territory. Any foreign invader to your territory is known as an "antigen," which triggers a violent response from your body. When your body comes into contact with an antigen, it reacts by rallying the troops—otherwise known as "antibodies"—within you to fight the enemy. The "fight" on your end is felt via your symptoms, which can range from minimal to extremely severe. With a food allergy, the battle you fight is not in your favor—going into shock as a result of fighting off peanut antigens is a classic example of a food allergy. Your castle has been terrorized and you're fighting with a vengeance.

Medically speaking, if you're allergic to a particular food, your blood will reveal the presence of immunoglobulin E (IgE) or antibodies because you are fighting the antigens within you—all of which is otherwise known as an allergic reaction. It's possible to have a wheat allergy, but this is different from wheat or gluten-intolerance; gluten-intolerance is *not* a food allergy, but a *delayed* battle or response from the immune system after the invasion has taken place.

To metaphorically illustrate *food intolerance*, consider the castle metaphor from a different angle. The invaders *capture* your castle. You were caught off guard and you didn't put up a fight, and now you're under siege for an extended period of time. In other words, you're in the enemy's hands. This can make you feel sick and produce one or more unhealthy complications, whereby the only way you'll feel better or heal is when the enemy leaves your castle, never to invade again, and peace is restored. For those with celiac disease or gluten-intolerance, there can only be a happy ending when the gluten-enemy is forever removed.

Who discovered that wheat was associated with celiac disease?

In 1888, celiac disease was first identified as a *wasting* condition associated with malabsorption. Dr. Samuel Gee of the United Kingdom's Great Ormond Street Hospital for Children documented cases of the disease in children, and aptly made a recommendation that diet would be a cure for the condition. Later, in 1953, William Dicke, a pediatrician from Holland, made the first association between celiac disease and wheat. He found there was an association between the protein found in wheat and the intestinal damage resulting from the ingestion of the protein. Dicke is credited with making the wheat-protein and celiac disease connection. But aside from these modern accounts of the disease, historical records reveal that humans have experienced digestive problems since 250 A.D. The Greek physician Aretaeus of Cappadocia studied individuals with a mysterious "suffering of the bowels," and referred to those afflicted as *koiliakos*. And from where does the word "celiac" originate? Centuries later, Francis Adams studied these accounts of Aretaeus and then coined those with the condition as "celiac," from the Latin version (*coeliacus*) of the Greek *koiliakos*.

Source: Celiac Sprue Association, A Brief History of Celiac Disease

Chapter 2

LIVING GLUTEN-FREE: WHAT ARE YOU IN FOR? REALITIES, EXPECTATIONS, AND PERSPECTIVES

- What is a gluten-free diet?
- What can you expect to learn from living gluten-free?
- How is living gluten-free like learning a different language?
- What is your level of gluten-intolerance or sensitivity?
- What can be done to make the transition to a gluten-free lifestyle easier?
- What are some advantages to living gluten-free?
- What are some particularly challenging aspects to living gluten-free?
- How much planning and preparation does living gluten-free take?
- Is a gluten-free diet restrictive?
- How vigilant do you have to be?
- What do you do when mistakes happen in following a gluten-free diet?
- What if you cheat on your diet?
- How sure can you be that you're eating gluten-free?
- How do you get out of the occasional gluten-free diet rut?
- What gluten-free publications can you subscribe to?
- Can you trust information on the Internet?
- How can a celiac disease/gluten-intolerance support group help you with your new lifestyle?
- What are the national support organizations for celiac disease and gluten-intolerance that have chapter affiliates across the country?

What is a gluten-free diet?

Diets often have a life cycle similar to fashion trends: They start off strong and gain widespread attention when driven by outlandish weight-loss promises, multi-million-dollar marketing campaigns, and often celebrity endorsements. Although appealing in the beginning, these diets eventually run their course, lose their popularity, show no sign of longevity, and are archived as the diet craze of a particular year.

Then there are other diets that are designed to be undertaken for a specific period of time to help correct a particular health issue, and once the goal is achieved, the diet is often modified or indefinitely shelved. But a gluten-free diet is different to either of these types. Neither a "here today, gone tomorrow" food industry phenomenon, nor a short-term corrective health measure, a gluten-free diet marks a dramatic shift in how we promote, regulate, and maintain good health.

Indeed, a gluten-free diet may be a matter of choice for those who say they feel better living without gluten, or at least less of it. But if you have to entirely eradicate gluten from your diet for medical reasons as prescribed by your doctor, the diet is not a choice. For those living with gluten-intolerance or celiac disease, the prescription or "cure" is a gluten-free diet, period. Following the diet is not optional, but mandatory and not just for a period of time, but for life. No need to despair, though! Your cure will not be malicious to the body, as other treatments for disease can be. In fact, it can bring new vitality to your life in ways you never imagined if you have an open mind, flexible palate, and positive attitude.

As a gluten-free diet becomes a way of life for generations to come, this relatively new way of eating will stand the test of time, continuing to make significant history along the way. So, what's ahead for you?

What can you expect to learn from living gluten-free?

When you embark upon the grand adventure of living gluten-free, your world will change in countless ways. First, you will probably experience a new profound sense of well-being once your uncomfortable symptoms disappear and healing within the body takes place. Not only will the core of your being, your gut, feel better, you may find that your mind feels healthier also—less brain fog, fewer headaches, clearer thinking. And what can you expect to learn from this improvement as a result of living gluten-free? Feeling sub par does not have to be a way of life! You don't have to wake up and feel bad and you can feel great after eating a wide array of foods. You can also expect to learn that you have control over how you feel by the food choices you make. Once on a gluten-free diet, you will never view food in quite the same light as you did before. In fact, you may never take food for granted again because you know how certain foods can harm you. A sobering realization. But, a new way of life is ahead of you with a broader awareness of your relationship with food.

Secondly, besides looking at food from a different perspective than you ever have before, your very actions and routines will change.

While the diet will seem challenging in the first several months, over time it simply becomes a part of who you are. You may even eventually forget what life was like before going gluten-free. Or at least, you won't care, because feeling better than you ever have will more than compensate for the efforts you make to stay gluten-free.

But in the meantime, venturing into the unknown is always helpful with a roadmap of realistic expectations at hand. When living gluten-free, you can expect all of the following to become aspects of your life:

- Being pro-active with and protective of your new-found well-being.
- Being aware of everything you eat, particularly with new foods.
- Reading food labels and packages ingredient by ingredient and looking for the GF symbol (the gluten-free designation) or allergen statements.
- Reading restaurant menus for gluten, asking questions of the staff, and doing your best to avoid cross-contact with gluten.
- Saying no to the gluten-based foods inevitably offered to you.
- Becoming a gluten educator. Explaining to friends, family, and colleagues what celiac disease or gluten-intolerance is and your personal experience with the condition.
- Educating restaurant staff about gluten.
- Being on the lookout for and researching new gluten-free products to add to your life.
- Satisfying your cravings with gluten-free foods.
- Broadening your world! Opening your mind and palate to new ingredients, recipes, tastes, and textures.
- Experimenting with new methods and techniques in gluten-free cooking and baking.
- Modifying your shopping habits and budget.
- Becoming accustomed to and delighted with the different flavors and textures of gluten-free foods.
- And last but not the least . . . feeling better, if not fantastic!

How is living gluten-free like learning a different language?

If you've always wanted to take up a different language, then now's your chance—but you probably never thought it would be the language of gluten-free food. The gluten-free lifestyle has its own unique lexicon, and in order to become well-versed in the art of gluten-free living, you'll have to expand your linguistics. But it's all in English, so no worries!

There are four distinct areas where you'll learn different words and phrases. They will soon become so familiar to you that you'll forget what life was like before you knew what they were.

GF Lexicon #1: Names for gluten
First and foremost, you will learn what gluten is, where it's found, and its many different disguises and derivatives. You'll learn you must avoid wheat, barley, rye, and possibly oats, and the importance of watching for "hidden gluten."

GF Lexicon #2: Ingredients on the "yes" list
These words will become more familiar as you read packages and work with recipes. They include simple names such as brown rice flour, tapioca starch, and sweet white rice flour, as well as typically unfamiliar names including teff, millet, sorghum, amaranth, manioc, xanthan gum, guar gum, and more.

GF Lexicon #3: Restaurant lingo
You'll learn the words cross-contact and cross-contamination and the subtle difference between them. And even though you don't have to become a chef, you'll need to become somewhat familiar with general cooking and baking methods and food preparation to steer clear of gluten on menus. For example, you'll always have questions about dusting and dredging while dealing with breaded and fried foods.

GF Lexicon #4: Cooking, baking terms, and techniques
You'll learn about "flour blends," in addition to a variety of other terms and techniques specific to gluten-free baking and cooking.

You'll need to archive what you know about traditional baking and learn a new methodology for success.

What is your level of gluten-intolerance or sensitivity?

Defining your level of gluten-intolerance or sensitivity is a critical piece of the puzzle for maintaining a gluten-free lifestyle. If you have been tested positive for gluten-intolerance or celiac disease, your tolerance to gluten is medically zero and there can be no deviation from the diet without producing a negative gluten response in your body. However, even if you have celiac disease, you must still determine your "reaction threshold" because, while trying to avoid gluten all the time as a prescription, some accidental ingestion of gluten traces might happen.

For example, based on how you feel after an incident of cross-contamination with gluten in a restaurant, you will quickly realize exactly *how* vigilant you must be in avoiding the cross-contamination possibility the next time you dine out. You'll also need to establish for yourself whether you can eat gluten-free products manufactured in a facility that also produces wheat products, or if your level of intolerance requires that you eat gluten-free products manufactured *only* in a 100 percent gluten-free environment. Your body will tell you when you've crossed the tolerance line.

If you are gluten-intolerant but do not have celiac disease, you may be able to get away with a little more trace contact with gluten than someone with celiac disease. You may be able to eat the top layer of a piece of pie (gluten-free filling) from the crust, but not be too worried should you ingest a few small crumbs of the crust. Find your limits and let them guide your decisions.

On the other hand, if you are only sensitive but not intolerant to gluten, your reaction-threshold will not be as severe as with the other two cases. Your level of sensitivity is based on your personal experience in consuming gluten and should be used to determine how much gluten you allow into your life.

What can you do to make the transition to a gluten-free lifestyle easier?

Taking on a lifetime responsibility of being proactive, careful, and wise in protecting your new-found well-being requires a strategic mindset. Without planning and effort up front, following a gluten-free lifestyle with ease won't be realistic. Expect a learning curve for at least the first three months, but if you know what to do in the beginning, the transition won't be as difficult. You'll find that when living gluten-free, thinking about where your next meal is coming from takes on a whole new meaning. But if practiced and implemented early on and regularly, the following rules will help you live the gluten-free lifestyle with relative ease.

- **Strategic Rule #1:** Think ahead, plan ahead. When you're traveling to visit friends and family, will they know what to serve you during a meal? What snacks will you bring with you that could possibly tide you over, if they must?

- **Strategic Rule #2:** Learn the language and know your subject. Do you know all of the ingredients you need to avoid? Do you carry cheat sheets with you?

- **Strategic Rule #3:** Whenever possible, have a plan B in mind. If you can't find a restaurant you can eat at when on a road trip, what will you do?

- **Strategic Rule #4:** Ask questions. When you are unsure, always ask, don't assume. Are you *sure* the chicken breast you ordered won't be dusted with flour?

- **Strategic Rule #5:** Think unconventionally. If the store-bought frozen gluten-free bread doesn't please your palate, perhaps gluten-free pancakes made from a mix or frozen waffles will work great for your sandwich slices.

- **Strategic Rule #6:** Form realistic expectations. Expecting the airplane to automatically have a gluten-free meal is unrealistic. Calling ahead to request a gluten-free meal is realistic.

- **Strategic Rule #7:** Know your possibility factors. The possibility of eating gluten-free at a fast-food restaurant is slim. The possibility of eating gluten-free at a health-minded restaurant is better.

What are some advantages to living gluten-free?

Even though the inherent challenges to living gluten-free seem overwhelming, you'll be delighted to know the numerous advantages far outnumber any difficulties you will find. It may be hard to recognize at first, but gluten-free living presents a world of abundance that is advantageous, delicious, and satisfying. But keep in mind you have to look for it too! While the advantages to gluten-free living abound and vary from individual to individual, always remember the adage: You get what you focus on. If you see lack and limitation with the diet, that is what it will be for you. Resolve to see the abundance in gluten-free living from the beginning, and your journey will be all the more advantageous.

- **Advantage #1:** If your body rejects gluten, the number one, hands-down advantage to living gluten-free is feeling better, if not immeasurably so. Lives have been dramatically transformed by following a gluten-free diet. Feeling good is priceless and living without gluten means living with so much more.

- **Advantage # 2:** Since a large majority of gluten-free products on the shelves are natural, organic, or simply less processed, living gluten-free has the power to guide you in making better, healthy choices consistently.

- **Advantage #3:** Sorry wheat, but it's not all about you anymore! Gluten-free living opens your world to a treasury of dietary staples, tastes, textures, and nutritious profiles you may never have otherwise discovered and experienced. A world of wholesome goodness, flavor, and satisfaction awaits you. You simply have to be open to what the adventure has in store.

What are some particularly challenging aspects to living gluten-free?

Adhering to the strict guidelines of any diet is challenging, and the gluten-free diet is no exception—it can be considered in many regards as one of the more challenging of them all. However, one of the secrets to meeting and overcoming challenges is knowing what they are in advance so they're not as surprising, and you can even turn some in your favor. You will encounter hundreds of challenges along the way, but just some of them include:

- Limited options. One look at a restaurant menu will very quickly drive home everything you can't have. The same scenario goes for grocery shopping. There's no reason to go down every aisle anymore.

- Saying no. Having to say "Sorry … none for me, thanks" when your server brings a basket of fresh bread to your table is a tough hurdle to get over, not to mention saying no to many other types of food you may be very accustomed to eating.
- Going cold turkey. No longer eating the foods you knew and loved. Missing some of those foods for which there are currently no gluten-free counterparts.
- Shopping cart envy. You can no longer put any food in the shopping cart just because it looks good. If it's not gluten-free, it stays on the shelf. Don't look at the other carts passing you by!
- Playing the game of "In Search Of." Finding stores in your area that carry a wide variety of gluten-free products you can eat. The smaller the city, the more difficult this can be.
- Dining out gluten-freely. Always carefully navigating restaurant menus and sometimes leaving a restaurant with virtually no options and having to find another. Avoiding cross-contamination with gluten will always be on your mind.
- Lack of spontaneity. Living gluten-free requires a great deal of thinking ahead and strategic planning so you don't go hungry or get sick. This constant mode of preparedness does not leave much room for spontaneity and letting the chips fall where they may when it comes to eating.
- Traveling. Finding restaurants that cater to you in even the strangest of places, and not always being able to eat the cuisine for which a country is well-known. Making space in already-crowded suitcases to bring food with you.
- Schools. Figuring out how to live gluten-free in college dormitories or making sure your child has a quality gluten-free school lunch.

How much planning and preparation does living gluten-free take?

When you adopt a gluten-free diet as a way of life, you can expect your life to change in several ways, one of which is the area of planning and preparation (P & P). Once largely taken for granted, regular activities of daily life such as eating, grocery shopping, dining out, and traveling now take on an element of premeditation. How much P & P gluten-free living will demand from you depends on your individual lifestyle. But you can expect to spend more time on it in the beginning, until you adjust and establish various routines.

Shopping becomes more methodical and not as spontaneous. Expect to give more thought to your grocery list than you ever did before, at least until you get the hang of finding what you can eat, planning your meals, finding recipes, and regularly purchasing the same products you like. You'll often linger in grocery aisles longer than you used to when reading labels. But on the bright side, your shopping excursions can become less time-consuming as you avoid certain aisles and head straight for those that provide what you need.

Regardless of experience, traveling will always require a fair amount of planning for all gluten-free lifers. From eating before going on a trip to bringing foods or snacks with you to researching restaurants in advance and ordering special meals on airplanes, traveling gluten-free takes on a new sense of time and personal responsibility.

Expect P & P to be bumped up several notches during the holidays, when socializing, and when letting family and friends know in advance how they can cook and bake for you when you visit.

In terms of time commitment, you can expect to spend hundreds of P & P hours over the course of your gluten-free life. But your health and happiness are worth it!

Is a gluten-free diet restrictive?

It would be untrue to say you won't find living gluten-free to be restrictive many times. It would be misleading to say that you'll never encounter challenges in finding something you can eat because you will, and it will happen more times than you can count. However, when going on a gluten-free diet, adopting a perspective from the start that focuses on options and abundance will do more for your success and happiness than looking only at what you can't have will do. Shifting to an abundant perspective despite the undeniable pockets of limitation and scarcity can be challenging indeed. But as many gluten-free diet pioneers will assert, modifying your perspective and opening your mind to different tastes and methods are a critical as well as enjoyable part of the journey.

To offer an analogy, consider the time-honored chocolate. You can find Hershey's Chocolate everywhere in America. But let's say, hypothetically speaking, you will never be able to eat the Hershey's brand again. What will you do? To replace Hershey's Chocolate, you'll find yourself searching for options. And when you discover and delve into a variety of sumptuous chocolate brands from Europe, your options increase and your indulgence factor soars.

Ladies, this type of scenario is also all too familiar when your favorite shade of lipstick has been discontinued and you're in search of a replacement. You typically find one you like even better, but may never have found that gorgeous shade had you not been forced into looking for it.

So, take a similar perspective with gluten. While gluten is indeed everywhere, when looking for other things to replace it, you'll find that your eating options will only increase and your variety factor improves as well. You can now look at other food staples with a new-found sense of appreciation and fresh approach to incorporating them into your diet. You will discover ingredients that are "new" to you but that have, in fact, been enjoyed by civilizations for centuries.

How vigilant do you have to be?

Vigilance is a word that conjures up effort; it takes physical effort and mental energy to be always awake and cautious about something that, should you deviate or relax for even a moment, could have very negative consequences. In the realm of gluten-free living, there is a universal law—your level of vigilance is directly proportional to your level of safety. The more vigilant you are, the more gluten-free you will be. If your vigilance varies unpredictably, your success in living gluten-free hangs in the balance.

If you have celiac disease, letting your guard down just once can be enough to get you sick. On a scale of one to ten, where one is low and ten is high, your vigilance *must* be a ten. Even though research suggests that minute traces of gluten may not be dangerous, your level of vigilance must be a ten because it will help you avoid making mistakes and ingesting levels of gluten that are unacceptable.

If you're gluten-intolerant, but not celiac, your level of vigilance should still be on the high end to avoid gluten, and it's up to you to determine how vigilant you want to be according to your own body and reactions. For you, ingesting gluten may be as uncomfortable as if you had celiac disease.

If you're gluten-sensitive, your level of vigilance will be determined by how important avoiding gluten is to you. If you know you're gluten-sensitive but are willing to put up with a fleeting and potentially embarrassing bout of gas that may come from eating your coworker's birthday cake (for example), your level of vigilance is relative to your desires at the time. Celiac disease does not allow for this kind of whimsical deviation. Those who are celiac or gluten-intolerant know the real meaning of having eyes behind their head and staying the course when it comes to avoiding gluten. But mistakes happen . . .

What do you do when mistakes happen in following a gluten-free diet?

The gluten-free lifestyle not only requires meticulous vigilance to keep you safe, it requires a realistic set of expectations, and experiencing occasional mistakes is part of the package. Even if you're following a book filled with tips, strategies, and guidelines for helping you avoid gluten 100 percent of the time, mistakes will still happen and you may feel sick as a result. Some mistakes will be more or less severe than others, but non-textbook, real-life experience will prove there is an inherent margin of error in living gluten-free.

Whether you're new to following a gluten-free diet or have mastered the protocol long ago, you're not immune to making a mistake or being a victim of a misunderstanding at some point on your gluten-free journey. Expecting that you will *never* encounter a cross-contact issue or accidentally consume some gluten is unrealistic unless you never eat outside of the parameters of gluten-free packaged products bought at the grocery store that are consumed in your gluten-free home.

Vigilance takes constant effort, and frankly, there may be a time when you let your guard down ever so slightly and make an assumption something is gluten-free when it is not. Or despite the best of intentions and high level of awareness from restaurant staff, something could be missed or explained inappropriately. Potential mistakes are numerous.

Accidentally ingesting a small amount of gluten will probably not result in a hospital visit, but it certainly can bring a flashback to how you felt prior to going gluten-free. If you have dermatitis herpetiformis, it might be advisable for your doctor to prescribe you the appropriate medication to have on hand in the event of an inadvertent brush with gluten and it can help relieve symptoms should an attack result.

Bottom line: Living gluten-free does not mean living risk-free. The only thing in your power is to limit your risk as best you can, learn from the mistakes you encounter, cope with the symptoms until they subside, and harden your shield with another layer of gluten-free vigilance.

What if you cheat on your diet?

The term "cheating" implies that you have consciously made a decision to break the rules of your diet and are willing to accept the consequences. Cheating on diets is common, and in fact, falling off the wagon and getting back on is a natural expectation when following a self-imposed diet. It's an inherent part of the process as you transition into a different phase of eating, whether it's a short- or long-term goal you're aiming for and whatever your reasons for the diet, be they losing weight or getting healthier. But for those who must follow a gluten-free diet for life to avoid severe physical implications, there is no lenience for cheating.

If you have celiac disease, any gluten you ingest will shift your body into attack mode to fight the evil invader (gluten), and in the process cause some level of damage your body will need some time to reverse. Even if you're gluten-intolerant but not celiac, cheating on the diet will also have its symptomatic implications that will take time to reverse.

The psychology of cheating takes on new meaning with a gluten-free diet. The mind-body association with gluten becomes so strong that the memory of feeling sick will often be incentive enough to avoid gluten at all costs, and conscious cheating will not be an enticing nor acceptable option for you. If you don't feel the pain associated with ingesting gluten because it is "silent" damage for you, your incentive to cheat needs to be stopped in its tracks. One way to help stop any thoughts of cheating involves vivid visualization. While you may not feel uncomfortable symptoms as a result of ingesting gluten, you must visualize the damage taking place within you. It's not a pleasant thought to envision how new, healthy villi in your intestine can become inflamed and flattened as a result of your noncompliance to the diet.

How sure can you be that you're eating gluten-free?

Naturally, one of the best ways to monitor whether or not you're gluten-free is how you feel, particularly if you're highly in tune with how your body reacts to gluten. If you're vigilantly following a gluten-free diet with accuracy, you can be fairly sure, almost 100 percent. But there may be times when you're just not certain. When you don't feel well, it's often natural to wonder if you consumed gluten somewhere or if you're simply experiencing similar, unrelated symptoms. It can be a time of confusion as well as frustration. Perhaps your vigilance steered a bit off course or someone inadvertently made a mistake in a restaurant.

However, living gluten-free is all about establishing realistic expectations, and there will be times throughout your life when you won't be 100 percent sure. But if you're following the strict guidelines without any deviation from the diet, you can be fairly sure you're eating gluten-free. Even if you experience a bout of illness associated with cross-contamination, you are eating gluten-free *overall* and that is what you should strive for.

As you follow the diet and begin to heal, your physician may order follow-up blood tests or even a biopsy after several months. The blood tests can provide you with a clear-cut scientific reading on how you're doing on the diet. Even with an isolated case of cross-contamination or noncompliance, your gluten antibody levels should be where they need to be if you're following a gluten-free diet closely on a daily basis.

How do you get out of the occasional gluten-free diet rut?

Ruts happen with all diets, particularly the long-term ones, and a gluten-free diet is no exception. In fact, a gluten-free diet can be more rut-prone than others because your options are inherently limited. In the beginning, a gluten-free diet is distinguished by exploration, discovery, and experimentation. You'll settle into a routine that is satisfying but after eating the same gluten-free foods over and over again (which you will!), boredom could strike and you'll be ready for new tastes. How do you get out of the rut or prevent yourself from getting into one? Consider the following examples:

Scenario #1: Gluten-Free Laundry

If your baked items, whether packaged or freshly made from a recipe, consist primarily of the "whites"—meaning flours and starches made from white rice, tapioca, and potatoes—it's time to switch over to the "colors" in the gluten-free spectrum; the brown, yellow, and golden colors. Look for flours with color and they will typically contain more nutrients and fun flavors than the whites. And if you're regularly eating white rice and potatoes, try making recipes using richly colored and nutrient-dense whole gluten-free grains. For both baking and cooking, search out products and recipes that incorporate colored grains and flours such as teff, quinoa, amaranth, buckwheat, mesquite, millet, and rich colored rice varieties such as black, red, brown, and wild.

Scenario #2: Musical Products
You'll typically discover one brand of pasta that is suitable to your palate, if not one that you really enjoy. But after eating the same pasta for the umpteenth time, you may be hungry for a creative take on the gluten-free pasta theme. While gluten-free pasta or noodles are commonly made from rice flour, search for pastas made with other flours such as corn, millet, buckwheat, and bean flours. Expand your versatility by using different shapes of pasta and new recipes. And when you get tired of the same gluten-free breads, cookies, and other baked delights, it's time to search out other options, find cookbooks, and experiment with different recipes to make your own in lieu of store-bought products.

What gluten-free publications can you subscribe to?

Although you may adore the glossy culinary and lifestyle magazines, they do not provide the gluten-free resource information you will need. Thankfully, there are two primary publications that specifically cover the gluten-free lifestyle. These magazines were the pioneers in covering the gluten-free diet beat and continue to remain on the cutting edge in providing timely news and support.

Gluten-Free Living

For over a decade, *Gluten-Free Living* has been a respected resource for providing helpful and thoroughly researched information for the celiac community about the gluten-free diet and lifestyle. The publication's advisory board, made up of leading physicians and dieticians in the field of celiac disease, provide their expertise to the publication. Founded by Ann Whelan, the publication has grown to a full-color magazine. For subscription information, visit www.glutenfreeliving.com.

Living Without

A full-color quarterly publication, *Living Without* is a lifestyle guide for those living with allergies and food sensitivities. Founded by Peggy Wagener, the publication continues to cover the gluten-free lifestyle from a wide variety of angles with articles, recipes, and information on cookbooks. The publication also offers an *Allergy-Friendly Dining Guide* featuring their favorite special diet eateries. For subscription information, visit www.livingwithout.com.

Can you trust information on the Internet?

If you've been around the Internet block, you know you have to read everything with one eyebrow lifted, always checking sources and taking much of what you find with a grain of salt. While it seems you can find an answer to virtually all of your questions with a simple run through a search engine, you're ultimately responsible for researching these answers and making the distinction between true fact or sheer fiction and everything in between.

You will no doubt use the Internet to find answers to questions that pop up along your gluten-free journey. And indeed the information you find can be fully credible, but much of it will indicate you need to keep searching. And always, always verify what you find with a reliable source.

Question Blogs

When looking for information about gluten-free living on the Web, be leery of blogs and chat rooms with people asking questions and getting answers from each other, particularly when they don't have credentials. These conversational venues can be mine fields of disinformation.

In the Name of Sale

Companies and storefronts can mislead you as they try to cash in on the gluten-free consumer. For example, any company site that promotes spelt as wheat-free and safe for the celiac diet is dead wrong. And there *are* sites that do this. Spelt *is* wheat, no matter how distant a relative it may be!

John GF Doe's Web site

Anyone can have a Web site, and there are virtually thousands of sites operated by individuals that claim to be experts on the gluten-free diet. And even though they have the best of intentions in sharing their knowledge and experiences with the online community, be careful, because the information may be inaccurate! Again, enter and review these sites at your own risk.

Your chances of finding accurate information exponentially increases when you visit established and respected resources, especially when medical information is needed. These resources include: a national celiac or gluten-intolerance support group headquarters site or chapter Web site; hospitals or respected medical/gastroenterology clinics; centers and associations such as the Mayo Clinic, National Institutes for Health, and the American Dietetic Association, or University centers such as the Celiac Disease Center at Columbia University or the University of Chicago Celiac Disease Program.

How can a celiac disease/gluten-intolerance support group help you with your new lifestyle?

It's comforting to know there's help when you need it most. And in the beginning stages of learning about and following a gluten-free diet, you may find that connecting with a support chapter near you can be beneficial in many areas. Even if you don't utilize an organization's services through a membership that usually comes with a nominal fee, just knowing they're there to help you when you need it is reassuring.

But as with any resource, it's optimal to know what they offer and how you can benefit. Below is a list of some of the many services and benefits you can receive by being a member of a national organization, a local chapter, or by simply visiting a professional organization's Web site.

- Guidelines for starting and following a gluten-free diet
- Lists of ingredients to avoid
- The latest news on celiac disease research, food labeling rules and regulations, the oats debate, and more
- Health materials and explanations of the condition and symptoms
- Lists of gluten-free products that have been researched and determined to be safe
- Lists of physicians and gastroenterologists in your area that specialize in celiac disease
- Lists of restaurants in your area that are gluten-free aware and offer gluten-free menus
- Lists of gluten-free cookbooks
- Gluten-free recipes
- Volunteer opportunities and new gluten-free friends
- Newsletters
- Special events, conferences, and food fairs
- Chapter meetings, classes, and more!

What are the national support organizations for celiac disease and gluten-intolerance that have chapter affiliates across the country?

There are a variety of organizations in the United State that can be useful resources for you, many of which have local support group chapters to join. They include

United States

American Celiac Society	www.americanceliacsociety.org	504-737-3293
Celiac Disease Foundation	www.celiac.org	818-990-2354
Celiac Sprue Association	www.csaceliacs.org	877-272-4272
Gluten Intolerance Group	www.gluten.net	206-246-6652
Raising Our Celiac Kids (R.O.C.K)	www.celiackids.com	858-395-5421

Canada

| Canadian Celiac Association | www.celiac.ca | 800-363-7296 |

Chapter 3

GLUTEN 101: DEFINING, FINDING, AND AVOIDING GLUTEN

- What is gluten? (Part One)
- What is gluten? (Part Two)
- Can proteins other than gluten be implicated in gluten-intolerance?
- Where is gluten found?
- Which foods commonly contain gluten?
- What grains, seeds, and starches are permitted, and which are not permitted?
- What are other names for wheat?
- What about spelt, again?
- Is buckwheat okay? It has wheat in its name!
- What's the scoop on oats?
- Are pure, gluten-free oats safe?
- What about malt?
- What is modified food starch?
- Is vinegar gluten-free?
- Is hydrolyzed vegetable protein (HVP) safe?
- Should you be concerned with rice syrup?
- Is vanilla extract gluten-free?
- What about caramel color?
- If something begins with "glut" as in "glutinous" does it have gluten?
- Is gluten found only in foods?
- Are alcoholic beverages and distilled liquors gluten-free?
- What does cross-contamination mean?

■ **What does cross-contact mean?**
■ **Is the glue used on envelopes safe?**
■ **Are laundry detergents gluten-free?**
■ **Is Elmer's Glue gluten free, and should you be concerned about paint?**
■ **Is chewing gum gluten-free?**

What is gluten? (Part One)

Before launching into the technical definition of gluten, it's interesting to note that this two-syllable ingredient is the subject of a counter-movement that is revolutionizing the way America eats and looks at food. And the majority of the population doesn't know it . . . yet.

Gluten can no longer be taken for granted as the primary ingredient it once was. This now-infamous ingredient has a reputation for being dangerous to a considerably large segment of the population in the United States, as well as other countries. Those who can't digest it can face grave physical consequences if it's not promptly removed from their diet. A pretty strong warning to be sure, but gluten's supreme reign in the food chain as an all-powerful and glamorized ingredient in cooking, baking, and product manufacturing is getting a run for its money. As the gluten-free diet continues to be the fastest-growing food movement in the United States, the role of gluten, or lack thereof, in the food chain is impacting the food industry and our lives as we know it.

With an increasing understanding of gluten and what it can do to the body, Americans are becoming more and more aware of their diet and their individual relationships with food. This modern-day gluten-saga continues to unfold, leading up to the undeniable conclusion that this one ingredient—found virtually everywhere we look—is not suitable for everyone, which raises several larger questions: Were our bodies naturally designed to tolerate gluten? As generations of families discover their intolerance to gluten, live life without gluten, and produce other generations who live without gluten, will this be a wake-up call to a new phase in human evolution?

So, then . . . what exactly is gluten?

What is gluten? (Part Two)

Gluten is a funny-sounding word, but it will become one of the most important words in your vocabulary. It sounds like glue, and it acts like glue. Most people, unless they are a chef or baker, don't know what gluten is. So, if you have never heard of gluten before, you're not alone. But this one word changes your life forever when you must avoid eating it. Get ready to be a gluten-buster!

Gluten is a storage protein found in several grains such as wheat, barley, and rye. Gliadin is the fragment of the gluten-chain that can't be digested by those with celiac disease or nonceliac gluten-intolerance. Gluten becomes sticky when moistened by other ingredients or the digestive juices in your body, and is naturally more difficult than most foods for the body to digest. Gluten helps hold things together. For example, the gluten in wheat flour helps give bread dough its viscosity and malleability, giving bread its structure and chewiness.

Wheat is the largest grain family and has many gluten cousins of different names, which you'll learn about. You'll need to look out for all members of the gluten-family tree.

While oats in their pure state do not contain gluten, they are often avoided because of cross-contamination with gluten, namely wheat, in the manufacturing process. Oats also have a unique protein, or peptide, that is believed by some to be similar to gluten. (See "What's the scoop on oats?" on page 59.)

Grains containing gluten are eaten whole and are also processed into flours and other substances that are used to make hundreds of thousands of foods around the world. As you begin your quest in avoiding gluten, you'll find that it's much like water: gluten is virtually everywhere. Gluten is sneaky and has many different disguises. If you don't look carefully, you will miss it.

Can proteins other than gluten be implicated in gluten-intolerance?

Gluten is the only protein known to be toxic to those with gluten-intolerance. Proteins found in other foods such as rice, corn, potatoes, meats, eggs, dairy, and gluten-free grains, for example, have no similarity to the gluten protein and are therefore safe. However, one protein that might be questionable for some is *prolamin avenin*, which is found in oats. While the oat protein is gluten-free and scientifically different from gluten, it is considered to have some similarities and has been found to be problematic to some individuals with gluten-intolerance and celiac disease. (See "Are pure gluten-free oats safe?" on page 60.)

Where is gluten found?

When you begin to search for gluten-free foods in grocery stores and restaurants, it soon becomes clear that gluten is at virtually every turn—not a comforting thought when your body is intolerant to it. In order to avoid gluten, you need to know what commonly contains gluten. So where is a good place to begin when looking for gluten in thousands of food products?

First, make the distinction between a natural, unprocessed food and a processed food. Unprocessed foods are foods in their natural state with nothing altered or added to them. These include foods such as fruits, vegetables, nuts, legumes, eggs, milk, fresh ground beef, or a fish filet. These foods are naturally gluten-free and you do not need to worry about them. On the other hand, processed foods have undergone a manufacturing process and often contain many different ingredients.

Rule #1: Virtually any processed or prepared food on the grocery shelf or in the deli section has the potential of containing gluten, so, be on guard.

Rule #2: If a food is packaged and has a list of one or more ingredients on the label, your gluten radar must be turned on and your label-reading skills will be put into action. (See "How do you read an ingredients list for gluten?" in Chapter Four.)

Rule #3: Anything that is made from flour is an immediate suspect for containing gluten. Processed foods containing flour such as breads, cookies, cakes, croutons, crackers, cereal, pasta, pitas, pizza crust, etc., probably contain gluten unless they are designated as gluten-free foods.

When you are at a restaurant, again, you need to know what contains gluten in order to avoid it. Grocery stores are excellent training grounds for learning how to read menus in restaurants. (See "What items on a menu should you be suspicious of?" in Chapter Ten.)

Which foods commonly contain gluten?

When walking the aisles of a grocery store or visiting a restaurant, nothing beats having a quick reference list of many different foods that commonly contain gluten. Some foods will even surprise you. "How can potato chips or French fries have wheat?" is a common question asked by baffled gluten-free beginners. One look at some varieties of Pringles Potato Chips with practiced eyes will reveal the hidden gluten (wheat starch).

The following list serves two purposes: first, to help you easily recognize where gluten *can be* and is *often* found; and secondly, to serve as a tool in finding gluten-free versions of those foods. The list may appear to eliminate nearly everything from your diet, but don't get discouraged. Virtually every food listed has a gluten-free version!

The following list provides a guide, but is not an exhaustive compilation. There are many other foods containing gluten that are not listed, and that is why reading labels is always imperative.

Baby food
Baked goods
Baking mixes
Breads, breading, bread crumbs
Broths and stocks
Bullion cubes and bases
Candy and candy bars
Canned soups
Cereals, cold and hot
Condiments
Crackers and croutons
Dairy products
Deli case foods
Desserts
Flavored coffee mixes and hot chocolate
French fries
Frosting
Frozen dinners
Gravy
Ice cream
Imitation meats such as crab meat
Licorice
Marinades
Pasta
Pizza crust
Potato chips
Processed cheeses

Processed meats
Protein drinks
Pudding
Snack bars
Salad dressings
Sauces and thickeners
Seasonings
Soups
Syrups
And the list goes on and on . . .

Remember: Any processed food can potentially contain gluten. To keep you cautious and safe take this phrase with you everywhere: "Everything is gluten-guilty until proven gluten-free." If a food is not inherently gluten-free, such as fresh fruits and vegetables, milk, eggs, nuts, pure butter, fresh meats, and so forth, you can't eat it until you investigate its gluten status and prove beyond a reasonable doubt that it's gluten-free.

What grains, seeds, and starches are permitted, and which are not permitted?

Civilizations around the world have developed and thrived on gluten-free grains and starches and have not made wheat the most pivotal ingredient in their diet, as North America and other countries have. So, it can be done; in fact, you'll probably discover and incorporate several foods you never have eaten before because you learned about them on the gluten-free diet. Get ready, your thinking is about to change, which is one requirement for living gluten-free.

First, let's look at what you *can* have. Mathematically speaking, you have more gluten-free staple options to choose from than you have gluten-based options.

Amaranth
Arrowroot
Beans (Legumes)
Buckwheat
Corn
Garfava
Job's tears
Millet
Montina
Nut Flours
Potato
Quinoa
Ragi
Rice
Soy
Sorghum
Tapioca
Taro
Teff

Now, let's look at what is NOT permitted on a gluten-free diet:

Wheat
Barely
Rye
Triticale (Hybrid of wheat and rye)
Contaminated oats

As you can see, there are considerably more gluten-free options. But because gluten-grains and their derived products are so prevalent in the American diet, you will spend a considerable amount of time trying to navigate your way around gluten. Once you get a good feel for what you must avoid, you can spread your wings and focus on what you *can* have, using the list of permitted grains and starches as a guide.

What are other names for wheat?

Wheat is the largest gluten family and comes in various disguises. This is where avoiding gluten can get tricky and mistake-prone if you're not at the top of your gluten-game. For example, semolina pasta is wheat pasta. In order to accurately maneuver around gluten, you need to know the variety of wheat-family costumes so you won't inadvertently open the door and welcome them into your gluten-free party.

The following list outlines various wheat-based names. Try to memorize these names because it will be helpful throughout your gluten-free living adventure.

Costume Name:	See-Through Hints:
Atta	Wheat-based / Indian flat bread
Bran	All-Bran Cereal
Bulgur	Often used to make tabbouleh
Dinkle	Another name for spelt
Durum	Wheat—read pasta labels!
Couscous	Made from semolina
Einkorn	Marketed as corn or maize, German wheat
Emmer	Another name for durum
Farina	Creamy hot wheat cereal; Malt-O-Meal
Farro	Another name for spelt
FU	Made from wheat, typically Asian
Graham	Graham crackers and crust

Kamut	Larger than wheat kernels
Matza, Matzo, Matzah	Traditional Jewish bread
MIR	Cross between wheat and rye
Semolina	Wheat—read pasta labels!
Seitan	Asian and vegetarian cuisine
Spelt	Often inappropriately labeled as wheat-free
Triticale	Hybrid of wheat and rye

Always watch for anything with "wheat" in front of it: wheat berries, wheat germ, wheat nut, wheat starch, and even wheat grass. The jury is still out on whether or not wheat grass is suitable for the gluten-free diet, particularly due to a possible cross-contamination issue in growing and harvesting. Do your research and consult with a physician or nutritionist before trying.

Resource: www.csaceliacs.org/gluten_grains.php

What about spelt, again?

Spelt is like a Halloween costume at a gluten-free party. It can appear to be gluten-free because it's sometimes inappropriately marketed as being safe for those with wheat intolerances. But on a closer look it's a gluten culprit. Spelt is a grain from an ancient wheat family of southern Europe and shares similar performance characteristics with wheat. While it does not have as much gluten parts per million as wheat, gluten is gluten regardless of the amount and spelt must be avoided on a strict celiac/gluten-free diet.

You may find spelt bread and other baked goods made with spelt flour labeled (inaccurately!) as wheat-free or even gluten-free, but don't let the labeling fool you. Spelt is a classic example of the necessity to know your gluten-ingredients and the many undercover names for gluten.

Is buckwheat okay? It has wheat in its name!

Again, names can be deceiving. Despite the "wheat" in its name, buckwheat is naturally gluten-free. Kasha is toasted whole-grain buckwheat, and buckwheat flour is often used in gluten-free baking. But now that you know buckwheat is gluten-free, don't become too smug at your discovery. There's a trap door you must avoid. For example, can you eat buckwheat pancakes? It depends. Investigate further because most buckwheat pancake mixes and menu items are made with wheat flour as the main ingredient. Buckwheat flour is merely added to impart its unique flavor.

See how tricky this can be. In your hunt for gluten, be aware of names and circumstances that can be potentially dangerous.

What's the scoop on oats?

Until recently, it's been recommended for someone with celiac disease and gluten-intolerance to avoid oats as strictly as they would wheat, barley, and rye. But some confusion still lingers—while you will still find oats on some lists of ingredients to avoid, you won't find them on others. This discrepancy raises serious concerns. For those not familiar with a gluten-free diet, the story on oats, the finer aspects of gluten-free lingo, and gluten-free grocery shopping, this can be potentially dangerous.

First, oats *do not* contain the toxic gluten protein per se. But, despite being scientifically gluten-free from Mother Nature's perspective, the primary reason why oats have been and continue to be blacklisted is because of the issue of cross-contamination with wheat in both agriculture and manufacturing processes. Most oats on the market are not 100 percent gluten-free, and are therefore unsafe for a gluten-free diet. It's extremely important to avoid popular oat brands on supermarket shelves as well as products containing oats that do not designate them as pure, gluten-free oats because of the strong likelihood of cross-contamination.

Until recently there has not been a pure, gluten-free oats product on the market for consumers to buy. However, pure, uncontaminated oats are now available. But the question is often asked: are pure, uncontaminated, gluten-free oats safe for the celiac diet?

Are pure, gluten-free oats safe?

Pure oats that are scientifically proven to be gluten-free are now available for the consumer to purchase. But questions have been presented about their safety for the celiac, gluten-free diet.

When you research the oats debate you'll find several national and international organizations have a position statement on oats, largely proclaiming their safety and describing their stance on including them in a gluten-free diet. Currently, it appears as though a majority of organizations have come to the consensus that pure, gluten-free oats are completely safe for the celiac diet, if consumed in limited quantity. However, it is advised that the small intestine be given adequate time to heal on a gluten-free diet before introducing pure, gluten-free oats back into the diet. Research suggests that from a quarter cup to one cup a day will not adversely affect individuals with celiac disease. In fact, a majority of organizations support their inclusion in the diet in the interest of providing high-quality fiber, other nutrients, and variety—a boon for those who love oats!

However, before you make your decision, it's important to note that oats contain another type of protein known as prolamin avenin that some people believe has characteristics similar to gluten. Even though research suggests that the majority can tolerate oats in small quantities, a small number of individuals with celiac disease react negatively to pure, gluten-free oats. As a result of this evidence, some individuals and organizations remain leery about including pure oats on the safe list until further long-term research provides the results they want to see.

If you decide to try pure gluten-free oats after thoroughly researching the issue for yourself, consider doing so carefully with small amounts under the supervision of your physician or dietician, and closely monitor how you react to them. Also, when consuming oats, discuss with your doctor if there is a need to take blood tests to monitor your antibody levels so that you have a biological green or red light to continue with oats.

While the debate about oats continues, it is nice to know that science reveals that oats are by nature gluten-free and when grown and processed in a 100 percent gluten-free environment they can offer yet another ingredient to enjoy and utilize for those who can tolerate them.

What about malt?

Once you think you have your gluten-free game down, it's not uncommon to reference the rule book occasionally because sneaky gluten-free vernacular can catch you off guard. Classic examples are foods that contain the word "malt." For example, ingredients such as malt, malt vinegar, malt syrup, malt flavoring, barley malt (both flavoring and extract), and malted milk contain gluten, because malt is a derived ingredient of barley. It's easy to assume that if you know malt is derived from barley, a gluten-grain, any ingredient that contains the word "malt" automatically contains gluten. But this is not necessarily the case.

One example is maltodextrin, a highly processed and purified ingredient that has a variety of uses in manufacturing food products. But maltodextrin can be derived from several different gluten-free ingredients that include corn, potato, or rice. It may also be derived from wheat. So, is maltodextrin gluten-free? North America typically makes maltodextrin from gluten-free starches, though it's commonly made from wheat in Europe. If you find maltodextrin on the ingredient list of an imported food from Europe, is it safe for you to eat? Scientific evidence sheds some light. Maltodextrin is so highly processed and purified that even the most scientifically sensitive and credible tests cannot detect gluten in maltodextrin. Yet, it's still recommended to be cautious with maltodextrin made overseas. In the United States, if wheat is used to make maltodextrin, the FDA requires the ingredient to be labeled "wheat maltodextrin."

What is modified food starch?

Modified food starch is an ingredient used by food manufacturers for a variety of uses such as thickening, stabilizing, emulsifying, and binding. Modified food starch is often found in foods such as soups, ice cream, salad dressings, pudding mixes, and frozen foods. As the name implies, the food is modified through a chemical process that creates desired physical properties like the ability to enhance viscosity or thickening performance, which the normal starch does not naturally have. It's also used as an anti-caking agent. For example, it's common to find modified potato starch in a can of mixed nuts.

But the term "modified food starch" has just enough ambiguity to raise eyebrows as to whether it's gluten-free or not, and can throw the unsuspecting gluten-free beginner off track. The word "food" in this ingredient should immediately raise a red flag, because it does not reveal what food is used in its name.

Fortunately, modified food starch in North America has a considerable degree of gluten-free safety because it's usually made from corn or potato and even tapioca. Plus, new food labeling laws require that food manufacturers disclose the source of the food used to make the starch. But, you must always be on guard for this ambiguous starch because it can be made from wheat. European countries typically use wheat starch. And Canada does not permit a product to be labeled gluten-free if it contains modified wheat starch.

Therefore, it's important to read ingredients lists carefully for modified food starch. If the product is made in America, you are probably safe, but may want to call the food manufacturer to confirm. If the product is imported from Europe and the ingredient label lists modified food starch, you will want to be more cautious because it will probably be made from wheat and won't be disclosed as the source on the label. And unlike research that suggests maltodextrin made from wheat renders the gluten undetectable, the process by which modified wheat starch is made is questionable in scientific circles. The modifying process can leave behind traces of gluten, and it's debated whether the residual gluten ppm (parts per million) is safe or not for the celiac community. Until further research is conducted, it's safe to avoid modified wheat starch whether you find it as an ingredient in a product made in the United States or find it listed as modified food starch in products imported from Europe.

Is vinegar gluten-free?

A variety of ingredients are currently overcoming serious image problems, and one of these is vinegar. Vinegars derived from non-gluten ingredients such as rice, apples (cider vinegar), grapes (balsamic vinegar), and wine are naturally gluten-free and are considered safe, while malt vinegar is not gluten-free.

However, distilled vinegar has often been blacklisted from the gluten-free diet. Foods containing distilled vinegar such as ketchup, mayonnaise, and mustard were commonly listed as foods to avoid in the past, and may still show up on outdated lists. But now these foods are being considered acceptable provided they do not contain any other gluten-derived ingredients that would bring the product into question. For example, a specialty mustard can contain distilled white vinegar but also wheat flour, making it not gluten-free.

Only until recently has distilled vinegar gained a place on the list of allowed ingredients for a gluten-free diet. And what is the reason for this change? Good old-fashioned science provides the answer. Indeed, distilled vinegar is derived from one or more gluten-grain sources, but it is believed that the distillation process effectively removes the gluten from the final product. Before this scientific reasoning came to the forefront, it had been commonly thought that gluten somehow could make its way into the finished product and produce a gluten ppm that could be unacceptable for highly sensitive individuals.

While science has determined that distilled vinegar is gluten-free, individuals can still be sensitive to it. However, the symptoms need to be attributed to something else, not gluten.

Tip: Check with manufacturers regarding fancy, flavored vinegars to rule out use of flavorings and processes that could make the product not gluten-free.

Is hydrolyzed vegetable protein (HVP) safe?

Also known as hydrolyzed plant protein (HPP), this mystery ingredient may be made from wheat, corn, or soy and will often show up in foods that require added flavoring such as gravies, sauces, and soups. Be watchful of this ingredient in restaurants that use pre-made mixes for making their foods. The FDA asks food manufacturers to disclose the vegetable or plant used, so if you see "hydrolyzed wheat protein" on the label you can put the product back. But if you see corn or soy in front of protein, it should be safe.

Should you be concerned with rice syrup?

Rice syrup is another ingredient to question. The "rice" in its name can lead you to believe that the ingredient is automatically gluten-free. But while most rice syrup used in North America is gluten-free as it's made from white or brown rice, barley malt enzymes may be used to manufacture this refined sweetener. And even though the gluten left behind may be negligible, you may choose not to partake. The best bet is to call the manufacturer to make sure the product is safe when rice syrup is listed in the ingredients.

Is vanilla extract gluten-free?

In the United States, vanilla extract is gluten-free. Whether the manufacturer uses grain or corn alcohol in the product, the distillation makes the grain alcohol gluten-free.

What about caramel color?

Carmel color made in North America is derived from corn. However, caramel color made in Europe is derived from wheat starch, but is considered gluten-free because it's so highly processed.

If something begins with "glut" as in "glutinous" does it have gluten?

When you're on a mission to avoid gluten, any word beginning with "glut" is enough to turn you in the other direction or at the very least cause suspicion because it looks similar to "gluten." But the majority of words beginning with "glut" are not associated with the forbidden ingredient. If you've wondered whether the "glutamate" in monosodium glutamate (MSG) has anything to do with gluten, you can be assured that it's gluten-free. And although "gluttony" means excess in eating or drinking, it has nothing inherently to do with gluten!

The one word that is the most suspicious of all is "glutinous," but there's no need to worry. While the word means having a similarity to glue, and gluten is glutinous because it has the quality of glue, glutinous is only an adjective and has nothing to do specifically with gluten. In fact, it's a word that can help you! Gluten-free baking relies on sticky ingredients to help ingredients bind together, improve texture, and add structure. Therefore, it's advantageous to seek out gluten-free ingredients that have a glutinous quality to them because they can add essential properties to a baked good. For example, glutinous is often associated with certain varieties of rice, like sticky white rice used for making sushi. Sweet white rice has a sticky or glutinous quality to it, and when turned into flour it becomes sticky when moistened and can help replicate the gluten-effect in baking. Other gluten-free flours, such as amaranth flour, can also take on a sticky or glutinous quality due to its high protein content. Glutinous can actually be a helpful word in your gluten-free vocabulary.

Is gluten found only in foods?

If you thought finding gluten in the foods you eat presents a trail of mystery, you'll soon discover the plot thickens when trying to find gluten in nonfood products. Finding gluten in products other than food requires close scrutiny, because gluten often hides out under ambiguous names in nonfood products and can easily throw you off the case if you are not methodical in its pursuit. Plus, other product manufacturers are not under the same regulations for ingredient disclosure as food manufacturers.

As gluten is like glue, it can help put and keep ingredients together that don't compose a food item. You need to analyze the ingredients of any product that comes in contact with your skin, particularly if you have dermatitis herpetiformis. Your skin is the largest organ and has the ability to absorb anything into the blood stream. Gluten is often used in shampoos, conditioners, and lotions for its protein value for hair and skin. You can find gluten in lipstick, other cosmetics, paint, and even Play-Doh! For more information on the debate about gluten in topical products, refer to Chapter Five.

Are alcoholic beverages and distilled liquors gluten-free?

Traditional beers, ales, and lagers are made from malted barley (gluten!), hops, yeast and water. These beverages are produced through a process of fermentation, not distillation, so they will contain unacceptable levels of gluten for a gluten-free diet and are blacklisted.

But even though a gluten-free diet may seem like a death sentence for beer lovers, there's reason to rejoice. Gluten-free beer, a relatively new, modern-day creation to hit the market, is an invention developed to meet the growing market demand for gluten-intolerant beer lovers. Gluten-free beers, lagers, and ales are typically made from fermented sorghum, buckwheat, and/or rice. The taste of a gluten-free brew is distinctly different from traditional beer, but is unique and not unappetizing. As the beer industry continues to take notice of the growing population of beer lovers adopting a gluten-free diet, more variations on the gluten-free beer theme are sure to be introduced by start-up entrepreneurs as well as the larger, well-known beer companies. (For a list of gluten-free brews, see "What are some brands of gluten-free beer?" on page 117.)

Other alcoholic beverages including whiskey, scotch, vodka, gin, and bourbon are made from gluten-grains but undergo distillation, which separates the gluten from the end product and renders them pure, gluten-free, and safe. Cordials like brandy and rum are also distilled and therefore gluten-free.

And wine lovers can rest easy because wine is naturally gluten-free, being made from grapes and other fruit infusions. Keep in mind that wine contains sulfates, which can produce sensitivities in some individuals, and if a flavored wine cooler incorporates barley malt it's not gluten-free.

As with any product, carefully read the label and if you have specific questions, call the manufacturer.

What does cross-contamination mean?

Gluten will fast become a vital word in your everyday vocabulary, and "cross-contamination" will be just as important as you navigate through a gluten-free life.

Cross-contamination occurs when a food that is otherwise gluten-free comes into contact with gluten, whether it's one gluten particle or a large amount. Cross-contamination can happen in three distinct areas: food preparation, food manufacturing, and agriculture.

The restaurant industry is a prime area for cross-contamination issues. If a gluten-based food touches a gluten-free food, cross-contamination has occurred and the gluten-free food is no longer safe. Any residual gluten left behind, even at the particle level, may make an individual ill when ingested.

There are countless ways cross-contamination can occur in restaurants; to illustrate, imagine that a pan used to sear a cut of meat dusted with wheat flour is then immediately used to sauté a plain chicken breast. Cross-contamination has occurred. The chicken breast is now contaminated with gluten and is therefore potentially harmful if eaten. Utensils are potential hazards also. If the same spatula used to flip wheat-based pancakes is used to flip your otherwise gluten-free fried egg, cross-contamination has occurred and your egg is no longer gluten-free.

Cross-contamination can also occur in the food manufacturing process. When wheat-based products share the same production equipment as products made without gluten and strict cleaning protocol is not in place, cross-contamination can occur. Even the slightest trace of gluten left behind on manufacturing lines can potentially cross-contaminate the gluten-free product. Many companies make only gluten-free foods and more such companies will certainly be founded to meet the growing need. For a listing of some strictly gluten-free dedicated companies refer to page 118.

Also, when crops are harvested next to each other or rotated throughout different fields, cross-contamination, or now being more commonly referred to as co-mingling, with a gluten-based crop can occur. This issue surrounds the oat debate.

And beware! Cross-contamination can occur in your own kitchen. Before you use any of your cooking equipment, read Chapter Five.

What does cross-contact mean?

Cross-contact and cross-contamination essentially mean the same thing and are often used interchangeably. Cross-contact happens when gluten comes into contact with a gluten-free food or when a piece of equipment, a utensil, or a fabric such as a hand towel has residual gluten left behind on the surface and comes into contact with a gluten-free food or your hands.

Using "cross-contact" versus "cross-contamination" is often a matter of semantics, but there is a subtle difference. Although cross-contamination is the most widely used of the two phrases, *cross-contact* best defines exactly what you want to avoid from the start: you want to avoid contact first, in order to avoid contamination. Without contact you can't have contamination.

In a restaurant there are hundreds of ways cross-contact can occur, and implementing strict procedures and standards for avoiding cross-contact is becoming paramount to servicing a growing population with special dietary needs. This serious issue requires a paradigm shift in thinking about food service operations among all service professionals, from chefs, cooks, and servers to dishwashers and bartenders.

Walt Disney World Resorts, for example, keeps ahead of the curve in developing cutting-edge service procedures and training practices for servicing guests with special dietary needs. Joel Schaefer, Disney's Culinary Development and Special Dietary Needs Manager, has the cross-contact issue down to a science which serves as a model for the hospitality industry to follow.

Is the glue used on envelopes safe?

In the United States, the sticky material used to seal envelopes is gluten-free because it's derived from corn or tapioca. However, this may not be true in other countries. To eliminate any concern, refrain from licking your envelopes and use an envelope sealer, glue stick or wet paper towel instead.

Are laundry detergents gluten-free?

As always, read labels and check with manufacturers for confirmation of gluten-free status. This will be of primary concern for those with dermatitis herpetiformis. Reading labels of soap and detergents can leave you scratching your head, so to jumpstart your search, all Unilever brands which include All and Surf contain no gluten and Proctor & Gamble consumer relations says that all of their laundry products are gluten-free. If you prefer natural-based detergents and soaps, Ecover's line is gluten-free except for their Lemon and Aloe dishwashing liquid.

Is Elmer's Glue gluten free, and should you be concerned about paint?

This is a particularly important question if you have children in school. Elmer's Glue is gluten-free, but their finger paints are not—they are made with wheat and oat products. Always inquire with the product manufacturer of any glue or paint used in your household or child's school to confirm what your family can and can't use.

Is chewing gum gluten-free?

It depends. Read the label; some gums are dusted with wheat flour to maintain freshness. It's recommended to call your favorite gum manufacturer to inquire about the gluten-free status of their gums and what kind of flour or powder they use to dust their gums. Wrigley's has a variety of gums that use granulated sugar in a form that looks like confectionary sugar. The company states they have a variety of gum brands that are gluten-free, some of which include Wrigley's Spearmint, Freedent, Doublemint, Extra, Big Red, and Orbit.

Chapter 4

READING FOOD LABELS: PUT ON YOUR SLEUTH HAT AND READ THE FINE PRINT

- What do you need to know about current labeling practices on packaged foods?
- How do you read a food package for gluten?
- How do you read the ingredient list for gluten?
- If a product label says "made in a facility that processes wheat . . ." is the food gluten-free and safe?
- If a package says "wheat-free," is it gluten-free?
- Does "no added gluten" or "no gluten" mean "gluten-free?"
- If a product doesn't say gluten-free and doesn't have any gluten ingredients, is it gluten-free?
- Does "gluten-free" on the package mean "100 percent gluten-free?"
- If a package says "all natural" or "organic," is the food gluten-free?
- When should you call a product manufacturer?

What do you need to know about current labeling practices on packaged foods?

If only *every* packaged food had a GF designation for Gluten-Free and a NGF designation for Not Gluten-Free, the lives of those living gluten-free would be immeasurably easier. However, because this is not the case and there is still much progress and enhancements to be made on gluten-free and allergen labeling regulations, learning how to accurately read food labels is a prerequisite for gluten-free living now and in the near future.

The decision to purchase a food depends on the information provided on the label by the food manufacturer, but if the information is not fully or accurately disclosed, how can you make the best, most informed purchase you can? Until recently, there have been no uniform recommendations or specific protocol by the United States government that guides manufacturers in how to accurately label their products as gluten-free. However, on January 23, 2007, the Food and Drug Administration (FDA) announced a proposed ruling on food labeling practices.

Without getting too technical about the language of gluten-free labeling regulations, the ruling currently provides the following criteria and new details and updates are expected to be unveiled in 2008:

- The definition of "gluten-free" means that a food or beverage has less than 20 ppm of gluten.
- For a food to be labeled gluten-free, it can not contain an ingredient from a "prohibited grain," which means an ingredient from any species of wheat, rye, barley or a crossbred hybrid of the grains such as triticale. But if an ingredient is processed to remove the gluten and falls below the 20 ppm threshold, it can be labeled gluten-free.

- A food will be considered "misbranded" if it does not adhere to the gluten-free criteria set forth in the ruling. Foods like milk and eggs that are naturally gluten-free cannot be labeled gluten-free. The ruling also suggests how a gluten-free claim by a manufacturer must be worded for foods containing oats or other foods that are by nature gluten-free, but still run a risk of containing gluten.

Reality check: Regardless of future labeling practices, you still need to become and remain a savvy consumer in the art of reading food labels.

How do you read a food package for gluten?

Label reading for gluten-free living is like brushing your teeth, checking the mail, or doing dishes—it becomes a routine. And if you have never read a food label beyond glancing at the calories and fat grams per serving information, your label reading prowess is about to become considerably more advanced. But take solace in knowing that it will become as natural as driving; you won't think much about it once you get the hang of it, but you'll always need the right keys.

Until more uniform gluten-free labeling practices are implemented and set in place over the next several years, product labeling will be inconsistent and you have to diligently inspect each product. Follow these two steps to exercise your label-reading muscles and to get a solid routine in place:

Step One: Look on the front of the package and in the product's title for the words "Gluten-Free" or the "GF" symbol. If you find one of them, you have immediate clearance to buy—almost. If not, go directly to the Nutrition Facts label on the package. It may be designated "Gluten-Free" at the bottom. Or you may find the heading "Contains," which will list any of the allergens in the product. If you don't see wheat or gluten, you have clearance (well . . . almost).

Step Two: If you can not readily find "Gluten-Free" or "GF" anywhere on the package, go to the ingredient listing usually found at the bottom of the Nutrition Facts box. You will find a laundry list of all ingredients in the product, and the basic rule of reading ingredients is: the ingredients are listed in the order of their amount in the product, most to least. Next step . . .

How do you read the ingredient list for gluten?

When you read a list of ingredients, you obviously start with the first on the list and work your way down to the very last ingredient. Keep in mind that you must make sure that every single ingredient on the list is gluten-free before you can purchase it. It's easy to gloss over words and miss something, but with label reading, you have to be very accurate or you run the risk of purchasing something you can't eat.

Start at the beginning of the list and look for any gluten-containing ingredients that should be avoided. Take the lists in Chapter Three to the grocery store with you for reference until you memorize the offenders. You will tend to look first for flour; you can be sure that "flour" is wheat flour. No gluten-free product manufacturer will list a gluten-free flour that way. They will be very specific, listing its full name such as brown rice flour, white rice flour, sorghum flour, quinoa flour or amaranth flour. If you see simply "flour," you can put it back on the shelf immediately. If you see "enriched" or "white flour" you can put it back. You can't assume "white flour" is "white rice flour" and they didn't put the "rice" in. Put it back!

If you don't see wheat, rye, barley, or oats, you still don't have clearance. If you see any of the wheat costume names such as "spelt," "bran" or "duram" put it back. If you don't, proceed with caution. After you have searched for the obvious culprits and don't find any, you've entered hidden gluten territory now. You will be looking for words such as malt, barley malt, wheat starch, oat flour, or soy sauce.

If after you read the full list, ingredient by ingredient, and do not see anything prohibited, do you have clearance? Not yet.

If a product label says "made in a facility that processes wheat . . ." is the food gluten-free and safe?

Product manufacturers that claim their product is gluten-free will often add a disclaimer on their label that says the product is manufactured in a facility that also processes wheat and perhaps other allergens such as soy, dairy, and tree nuts. The purpose of this disclosure statement is to let consumers know the full range of products their facility produces so they can make a well-informed decision about whether to buy the product or not, as well as to limit the manufacturer's liability. So, is the product safe? The product itself can be naturally gluten-free or made with all gluten-free ingredients, but the statement acknowledges the possibility of cross-contact with gluten.

Some manufacturers will take every precaution necessary to thoroughly clean the equipment that processes ingredients containing gluten before they switch over to process the gluten-free product. Some manufacturers may not be as careful. To help answer how safe or tolerable this "gluten-free" product may be for you, you need to know your level of gluten sensitivity. If you are highly sensitive and may have a reaction to something as small as gluten-particle dust, you may decide not to buy the product. But if you can get away with a minute trace of gluten without a reaction, you're probably okay.

It is not uncommon for natural food stores to put this disclosure statement on foods like dried fruits and grains that they have purchased and repackaged, many of which are by nature gluten-free.

Therefore, to define the product's level of safety for you, consider calling the product manufacturer or store directly to ask them whether and how they clean their equipment before making or packaging the gluten-free product, and whether they can tell you what their gluten ppm is in random batch testing. Based on their answer, you can choose whether to buy the product or not.

If a package says "wheat-free," is it gluten-free?

For the gluten-free living apprentice, the "wheat-free" label can be a trap. This is a classic example that illustrates the importance of understanding gluten-free semantics. "Gluten-free" automatically means "wheat-free," because a gluten-free product cannot contain any ingredient derived from the species of wheat. However, "wheat-free" on a package that does not also specify "gluten-free" does not necessarily mean the product is gluten-free. For example, a product containing rye or barley but not wheat can be legitimately labeled wheat-free, but it is not gluten-free. Also, many products using oats but not wheat are often labeled wheat-free, but as the cross-contamination issue continues with oats, you must base your decision to buy this product on your known tolerance level of oats. If the oats are not pure, gluten-free, the product will not be gluten-free because of the likelihood of cross-contamination with wheat.

Then what about wheat-free soy sauce or tamari? Typically, traditional soy sauce is made with wheat and contains gluten. But soy sauce is not made with rye or barley. So, if a soy sauce brand says "wheat-free" but not "gluten-free," you can be sure it's gluten-free as well. This may sound contradictory to the information just stated, but again, it's important to know your gluten-based and gluten-free ingredients to understand products accurately.

Caution: Some baked products utilizing spelt (a species of wheat) have been misbranded in the past as "wheat-free." You may still find misbranded products in small independent stores and bakeries. It's not uncommon to find bakers and other product manufacturers who are unfamiliar with the gluten-free diet and its labeling protocol, and think spelt and other wheat-related grains are wheat-free. A search on the Internet will reveal numerous companies that inappropriately claim that spelt is wheat-free.

Does "no added gluten" or "no gluten" mean gluten-free?

Gluten-free linguistics can get a bit tricky when defining authentic gluten-free status. While food manufacturers must adhere to strict guidelines in labeling products as gluten-free, the "no added gluten" tag is becoming more prevalent in the food service and product manufacturing niches as a protective measure that essentially can mean the same thing as "manufactured in a facility that produces products made with wheat." The term "no added gluten" can mean that a product is made with gluten-free ingredients and nothing containing gluten has been physically added to the product, but it does not necessarily mean it's gluten-free because there is the potential of cross-contamination. Putting this tag on the product does not make them liable for a gluten-free claim.

If a product was made in a restaurant or bakery, the "no added gluten" means they can not guarantee that gluten particles in the air from pastry dust, for example, did not come into contact with the gluten-free bread batter. If you see the "no added gluten" term, it's up to you to make the final decision whether you will partake or not.

For restaurants that would like to create gluten-free menus for their customers but can't guarantee a 100 percent gluten-free environment, it's wise for them to add the "no gluten added" phrase to their designated menu items so customers can easily recognize meals without gluten ingredients. As more restaurants jump on the bandwagon and adopt this phrase, it indicates that awareness is improving and the industry is headed in the right direction—an equation that means more gluten-free options for gluten-free diners.

If a product doesn't say gluten-free and doesn't have any gluten ingredients, is it gluten-free?

Good question. The answer is maybe. Keep in mind that a company can voluntarily label its product gluten-free according to new FDA guidelines, but is not required to do so. If it's not labeled gluten-free, one of the following reasons may apply:

Reason #1: While all of the ingredients in the product are gluten-free according to Mother Nature, if the product is shared with equipment that processes wheat or gluten, it could be cross-contaminated and yield a gluten ppm test result that is more than 20 ppm. This would prohibit the company from labeling the product as gluten-free. This measure is in place to protect you, because a higher-than-acceptable ppm could make you ill. And even though some companies test their products for gluten ppm and consistently come underneath 20 ppm, they may not want to take the risk. Choosing not to label their product as gluten-free will limit their liability despite the possible drawback of fewer sales.

Reason #2: The company has not yet sold all of its old, outdated packaging that is not labeled gluten-free, and until the old inventory is sold, you won't see their newly gluten-free label on the shelves. If it's a product you really want to try but are unsure, keep watching the packaging or call the manufacturer for a confirmation.

Reason #3: The product could be a singular ingredient that is inherently gluten-free such as milk, eggs, pure butter, or canned green beans in water. But according to new labeling regulations, a company would be "misbranding" their product by labeling it gluten-free. Know your singular, inherently gluten-free foods so you don't have to worry about reading labels and proceed quicker to check-out!

Does "gluten-free" on the package mean "100 percent gluten-free?"

Not necessarily. But don't get discouraged! A gluten parts per million threshold is in place. According to the proposed Food and Drug Administration's definition of gluten-free, a product cannot be labeled gluten-free unless its gluten ppm threshold is 20 or less. So, mathematically speaking, if a product tests at 20 ppm it's obviously not 100 percent gluten-free, but is gluten-free enough to be safe. The ppm is so negligible that anything at or below 20 will, in most cases, not adversely affect even the most sensitive person. Therefore, it's safe.

For example, distilled vodka made from grain alcohol is considered gluten-free if its ppm rating is 20 or below. While a prohibited grain was used to make the vodka, the distillation process renders the gluten harmless. The scenario applies to distilled vinegar as well. While it is derived from a gluten-based grain, the product becomes gluten-free through distillation and is considered safe.

Gluten-free products are closest to being 100 percent gluten-free when they are made in a 100 percent gluten-free manufacturing environment and when all of the ingredients used are 100 percent gluten-free. Without gluten particle dust in the air, a product's ppm will be as low as it can get from a manufacturing environment perspective.

You will come to recognize the tried and true gluten-free brands that are highly respected in the industry. And chances are very slim that a company will misbrand its product as gluten-free to capitalize on the gluten-free market demand. The possible legal repercussions are not worth the risk. But, as always, it's important to be aware of a company's reputation and if in doubt, call to inquire about their manufacturing practices, ppm testing procedures, and results.

If a package says "all natural" or "organic," is the food gluten-free?

When you adopt a gluten-free lifestyle you'll don several hats, one of which is "label reader." But you probably never would expect the gluten-free life would also begin with a crash course in marketing and advertising lingo. Not only do you have to know how to look for and avoid gluten, you need to learn packaging linguistics as if you didn't have enough on your plate.

The two most commonly used terms in the world of product packaging are "all natural" and "organic." While these words are blessings for those who enjoy a healthy lifestyle, they are umbrella words that describe the overall nature of a product and can trick the unsuspecting gluten-avoider. If a product is coined "all natural," it does not use unnatural ingredients. If a product is coined "organic," it's made with ingredients grown and manufactured according to strict organic regulations. Some products are just partially organic, utilizing organic ingredients when they can.

A large portion of gluten-free products are labeled "all natural" or "organic," but don't assume that all foods with those labels are gluten-free. You have to research the product further. A person unfamiliar with the health food industry may come across many unfamiliar terms, such as "All Natural," "Organic," "Hormone and Pesticide Free," "naturally raised," "cage-free," and many more. It may seem as if they all blend together and mean the same thing. But a lesson in natural food terminology quickly reveals that each term has its own distinct meaning. While you may like the words "all-natural" and "organic," you can't stop there. You must always look for the words "gluten-free" or at least analyze the product to make sure there's no gluten, whether or not it's labeled "all natural" or "organic."

When should you call a product manufacturer?

You may feel the need to call a company at some point to inquire about the gluten-free status of one of their products. There are cases in which you should call just to verify the gluten-free nature of the product, and there are times when you must call before you ingest something. As you journey through your gluten-free life, you may want to call because:

Case #1: You find a product that appears to be gluten-free by the nature of the ingredients they use, but nowhere on the package can you find a gluten-free designation. In this case, you may want to call to ask them about their manufacturing processes. Does this product share the same production lines with wheat? Do they test for gluten, and if so, what are their ppm results? Remember, not all gluten-free products will be labeled gluten-free because it's up to the manufacturer to do so.

Case #2: If you tried a product you believed to be safe and you did not feel well after eating it with symptoms that mimicked a reaction to gluten, you should consider calling to ask about their manufacturing process or see if you missed any hidden gluten. This can help determine if you will purchase the product again or not.

Chapter 5

THE KITCHEN: MAKING YOUR KITCHEN GLUTEN-FREE

- How do you make your kitchen gluten-free?
- Where does gluten hide in your kitchen cupboards?
- Where does gluten masquerade in the refrigerator and freezer?
- Should you throw away the toaster, and what about the oven?
- Are your pans, utensils, and cutting boards safe?
- How should you store your gluten-free flours and grains?
- Are kitchen soaps and cleaning products gluten-free?

How do you make your kitchen gluten-free?

Making your kitchen gluten-free all begins with getting rid of the old and making room for the new. Start with the pantry and cupboards. Remove all food and nonfood products from the cupboard, placing them on the counter so you will have a completely empty cupboard to clean. Thoroughly wipe down all shelves with warm soapy water, removing all crumbs (gluten!) or sticky residue from bottles and sauces. Let dry. With a clean cupboard and pantry you're now ready to begin sorting through the products you can keep and setting aside those you can no longer eat or use. Analyze each food to determine its gluten-free status using your label reading skills from Chapter Four. Any products in question need further investigation before being granted reentry into your cupboard! Follow the same process above for your refrigerator and freezer.

Now, make a list of the products that did not pass the test of entry into your new gluten-free cupboard and refrigerator. This will begin your restocking phase. Based on your list, find and buy the gluten-free versions of those foods to replenish your kitchen. Refer to Chapter Six: Food Products: What Are Your Options? for tips on gluten-free brands.

But you're not done yet. You must thoroughly clean or eliminate equipment and utensils that have been used to handle gluten to ensure safety from cross-contamination before you are in full operation again.

If you're the only one in the household eating gluten-free, designate cupboard and refrigerator space for your gluten-free foods to keep them separate from the gluten-based foods your family eats. Also, be sure to designate equipment, utensils, and storage containers as gluten-free and store them in an area that does not share space with equipment that does have contact with gluten.

Where does gluten hide in your kitchen cupboards?

When making your kitchen gluten-free, you will find yourself eliminating a variety of foods right off the bat as obviously gluten-guilty. These foods typically contain wheat flour as their main ingredient, such as all-purpose wheat flour, breads, cereals, pancake and biscuit mixes, cake mixes, cookies, crackers, and pasta. Wheat flour is generally listed as the first ingredient, making them easy to eliminate at first glance.

On the other hand, there will be many foods that are not as easily recognizable as containing gluten and you will need to read the label further. These types of foods include soups, sauces, broths, spices, flavorings, seasoning packets like taco seasoning, drink mixes, candy bars, potato chips, beverages, and many more. Always remember that any processed food that contains more than one ingredient is an automatic suspect for hidden gluten. You have to look at everything!

Also, don't let brand names fool you—they can be gluten decoys. For example, Rice Chex cereal is not made just from rice, it has wheat flour as the main ingredient. Be watchful of things like Corn Bread mix also. While it may appear initially that the product is made from corn, the name is deceiving and again you will often find the first ingredient listed is wheat flour. Never assume!

And it can get even more mysterious. Have you checked your tea lately? Many teas have other ingredients besides tea leaves like barley (gluten!) often used as a flavor enhancer. Who would have suspected?

Where does gluten masquerade in the refrigerator and freezer?

You can't let cold foods fool you. To eliminate the gluten in your refrigerator and freezer, use the same clues you used when finding it in the cupboard—cold gluten can be just as tricky to find.

Save time by not investigating the raw, unprocessed, naturally gluten-free foods in your refrigerator such as fresh fruits and vegetables, eggs, milk in the carton, and fresh meats. You can then quickly eliminate foods such as bread, frozen pizza, cookie dough, pie crusts, dinner rolls, and leftovers made with the gluten-containing ingredients found in your cupboard, things like spaghetti and macaroni and cheese.

Other foods are not as easy to recognize. Investigate your salad dressings, condiments, sauces, all frozen dinners, pancake syrup, French fries, processed meats, sausages, and even take-out leftovers from the neighborhood Chinese restaurant. And like Rice Chex in the cupboard, watch out for ingredients where their first name is a decoy, such as soy sauce. The other ingredient in soy sauce besides water is not soy—it's wheat!

And if you never thought dairy could contain gluten, think again. Hidden gluten can be found in dairy-based foods such as ice cream, sour cream, cottage cheese, margarine, yogurt, cheese, creamers, and whipped cream. Be even more careful with non-dairy items such as creamers, coffee flavorings, and processed cheeses. Remember, the more processed and unnatural the food, the higher the risk that it contains gluten.

Finally, look at every beverage! Beer is made from wheat and barley malt, and many canned sodas and beverages made from powdered mixes can contain hidden gluten.

Should you throw away the toaster, and what about the oven?

If there is any piece of equipment in the kitchen that needs your immediate attention, it's the toaster. Toasters are catch-alls for gluten crumbs built up slice after slice, not to mention they are cumbersome to clean. Opening the hatch door to release the crumbs is a start, but typically crumbs and gluten-residue will still be hiding throughout the toaster, often visible on the walls and in hard-to-clean corners. Unlike a conventional oven, a toaster can't produce the high heat necessary to kill residual gluten left behind—you are better off replacing your toaster with a new one. Chances are likely your toaster is ready for a replacement anyway! And don't forget to keep in mind that you always need to watch out for toasters away from home when visiting family or restaurants.

Toaster ovens and microwaves must also be thoroughly cleaned. Remove all racks and trays to thoroughly sanitize them, using a bit of steel wool if necessary to eliminate hard-to-remove build-up. Scrub the inside of the oven, paying close attention to the walls, ceiling, door, and window. Leave no trace behind, or you'll need to replace the oven!

Also, it's common to be fearful of using your conventional oven when you know you have baked many foods laden with gluten, but you need not be. Simply clean your oven thoroughly as you would normally, paying especially close attention to removing caked-on matter. For added safety, set the oven temperature at 500 degrees Fahrenheit and let it bake for fifteen minutes to kill any gluten that may be left behind after cleaning.

Finally, clean your stove surfaces, making sure to remove any possible trace of gluten resulting from pots that boiled over or spilled crumbs. Knowing everything is as clean as possible will give you peace of mind.

Are your pans, utensils, and cutting boards safe?

Don't worry—you won't have to throw everything away. You will, however, need to follow some basic guidelines to ensure your safety from prior contamination with gluten.

Any piece of equipment or utensil in your kitchen that has come into direct contact with gluten has to be either thoroughly washed or thrown away. The kitchen abounds with cooking and bakeware made from materials ranging from smooth, easily washable surfaces like stainless steel, glass, and hard plastics, to more porous surfaces like Teflon, wood, and soft plastics. Anything can trap gluten.

Stainless steel pots, pans, and silverware can be easily washed and sanitized under very hot water and dish soap or in the dishwasher. Typically, any residual gluten that may have been left behind—say by boiling a pot of pasta for the non-gluten-free members of your family—can be cleaned away, rendering your equipment safe to use.

On the other hand, Teflon surfaces on skillets and pots are tricky because nicks and chips in the surface leave behind crevices where gluten particles may be trapped. This equipment can be questionable even after thorough cleaning.

Also, be watchful of bakeware that has any post-baking matter, like the familiar black, crusty glue that sticks to rims and corners and does not wipe away easily. This crusty gluten build-up must be removed entirely to ensure your safety. You may find some of your equipment is beyond thorough cleaning and needs to be thrown away or replaced.

Be extra cautious of cutting boards, waffle irons, spatulas, wooden spoons, rolling pins and anything else with corners, cracks and crevices that can trap gluten particles. Also, thoroughly wash dishrags, hand towels, hot pads, and mittens. Remember: When in doubt, throw it out.

How do you store your gluten-free flours and grains?

Gluten-free flours are expensive, and if you like to cook and bake from scratch, you'll want to pay close attention to protecting the shelf life of your flours as long as you can. Always keep flour away from direct sunlight or moist air. Storing flours in dark, dry places like cabinets is better for their longevity than keeping them in fancy, clear glass canisters on the counter where light can penetrate them.

Upon opening, it's best to refrigerate certain gluten-free flours to protect taste and texture as well as extend their life. Those that have high fat content are prone to rancidity and should always be refrigerated. These include flours such as nut flours, flaxseed flour, amaranth flour, brown rice flour, and millet. If you live in a warm and humid climate, refrigerating your flours is recommended regardless of flour type. However, always refer to the directions on the package.

Whether stored in the refrigerator, freezer, or cabinet, make sure your gluten-free flours are well protected from air; simply rolling down the package and clipping it with a clothespin is not going to produce an airtight environment. Consider transferring them to plastic containers with lids or durable plastic bags, like heavy-duty freezer bags. But if you choose to use the packages that the flours come in, at the very least, double protect them by placing them inside food-quality, plastic storage bags and sealing them tightly. These storage tips are also applicable for your gluten-free grains such as teff, quinoa, and amaranth.

Are kitchen soaps and cleaning products gluten-free?

As with food and medications, cleaning products can harbor hidden gluten. Therefore, always read product labels and confirm with the product manufacturers when you have questions about gluten-free status. Remember: Anything is gluten-guilty until proven gluten-free and ingredient labels can change so continue to monitor them. To save yourself some time and possible aggravation, refer to a variety of gluten-free cleaning products found in *The CSA Gluten-Free Product Listing* published and regularly updated by the Celiac Sprue Association's national headquarters. This comprehensive compilation has done the research for you. Just some of the companies listed that have gluten-free products in their line include Ajax, Palmolive, and Seventh Generation.

Chapter 6

FOOD PRODUCTS: WHAT ARE YOUR OPTIONS?

- What are some tips for stocking a gluten-free kitchen?
- What can you expect from gluten-free breads?
- What are some gluten-free bread recommendations to get started?
- What are some brands of packaged gluten-free breads already sliced?
- What are some brands of gluten-free bread mixes?
- What are some brands of gluten-free pasta and noodles?
- What are some brands of gluten-free all-purpose flour blends for wheat flour substitution?
- What are some brands of gluten-free baking mixes?
- Who supplies individual gluten-free flours and starches?
- Who are some suppliers of gluten-free grains?
- What are some brands of gluten-free cereal?
- What are some brands of gluten-free oats?
- What are some brands of packaged, ready-to-eat cookies, biscotti, brownies, and other baked delights?
- What are some gluten-free snack bars and nutrition/energy bars?
- What are some brands of gluten-free frozen meals?
- What are some brands of gluten-free crackers?
- What are some brands of gluten-free potato chips?
- What are some brands of gluten-free soy sauce and other sauces?
- What are some brands of gluten-free beer?
- What about soy milk and rice milk?
- What are some companies that have 100 percent dedicated gluten-free facilities or dedicated equipment for certain gluten-free products?

What are some tips for stocking a gluten-free kitchen?

Bewilderment is a natural reaction when first charged with the task of finding gluten-free replacement foods. But as you become more familiar with various gluten-free brands on the market, as well as beginning to think outside the box to come up with your own alternatives, your kitchen will become a well-stocked place that serves your needs nicely.

To get started, think about your eating habits and cooking needs before going gluten-free. If you like to primarily bake and cook from scratch, your needs will be different than if you prefer to bake and cook using prepared foods and mixes. Like most people, if you do a combination of both, your kitchen will need to support both aspects.

Following are some ideas for stocking your kitchen in the beginning:

- Keep gluten-free pastas on-hand for convenient meal preparation. They come in a variety of different shapes to make virtually any pasta dish you were accustomed to.
- If you like pancakes and waffles, there are a variety of gluten-free mixes on the market that are extremely versatile. Some mixes make pancakes as well as cookies, muffins, crepes, and scones. If you like cereal, you can find both hot and cold versions widely sold in natural food markets.
- Have a collection of individual gluten-free flours on-hand, such as brown rice flour, corn starch, and arrowroot starch, to replace wheat flour when you want to thicken gravies and sauces. If you like to bake, of course you will have to stock your kitchen more thoroughly with a variety of gluten-free flours, starches, and baking aids (see Chapter Thirteen).
- Gluten-free breads can be made from mixes or purchased in loaves, often found in the freezer section of natural food markets.

- Stock your refrigerator with gluten-free salad dressings, and have gluten-free packaged snacks available in the cupboard such as cookies, crackers, and breakfast bars.

What can you expect from gluten-free breads?

Whether you're shopping for or baking gluten-free bread, get ready for your thoughts on and expectations of bread to change. The differences will surprise you—if not annoy you—at first. But with time and practice you'll discover the breads you like most and will build loyalty to certain brands and recipes, slowly becoming accustomed to the inherent differences between wheat and gluten-free bread.

Difference #1: Shopping.

While options for purchasing traditional wheat-based loaves are abundant and cost efficient, you'll quickly find that you have fewer gluten-free bread options and they're considerably more expensive. Shopping for gluten-free bread takes a sense of research, effort, and experimentation. You'll find that most gluten-free breads are located in the frozen food section. They will be smaller, heavier, and often quite dense. Also, expect your bread budget to increase, particularly if you continue to eat as much bread on a gluten-free diet as you did before it.

Difference #2: Baking.

There are two kinds of gluten-free breads: quick breads (breads made from batter that is leavened with baking soda or powder instead of yeast) and yeast breads, both of which resemble cake batters and are baked in loaf pans with walls. With gluten-free breads, say good-bye to kneading. You can't knead a gluten-free batter, but you will mix it like you would a cake.

Difference #3: Taste and Texture.

Generally speaking, you will find that most gluten-free breads taste and feel different than wheat flour-based breads. Some gluten-free breads will be dry and crumbly, while others will surprise and delight you with a moist and spongy quality. Experiment with different types, recipes, and brands to find a gluten-free bread that you like.

Reality Check: Like shopping for cosmetics—which you often purchase, get home, and hate—shopping for bread options will probably yield similar unusable results. Explore and experiment with a patient attitude.

Key Expectation: Typically, you can't leave gluten-free bread out on the counter for days like you can traditional bread. Most gluten-free bread is usually best kept frozen and eaten by the slice as you need. Plus, it doesn't have the preservatives that shelf breads have. And say hello to the toaster! You'll be toasting many a slice to enhance texture as well as flavor.

What are some gluten-free bread recommendations to get started?

Finding good gluten-free breads can be challenging, particularly if you're looking for them for the first time. To get started, you have five basic approaches to research and try.

Option One: Make a Beeline to the Freezer Section.

When time is of the essence or if you don't want to bake your own bread, you can investigate pre-made gluten-free breads that are pre-sliced and found in the freezer section of most natural food stores.

Recommendation: Food For Life, a manufacturer of organic grain bread, has a fairly wide line of gluten-free breads featuring different whole grain rice flours including brown, red, and black rice versions.

Option Two: Find a Bakery.

Research bakeries in your area for fresh-baked gluten-free breads. The availability of gluten-free bakeries varies dramatically from state to state, but it's worth a try no matter where you live.

Recommendation: Many bakeries in other cities will ship to your address, so don't get discouraged if there isn't a gluten-free bakery in your city.

Option Three: Mixin' Magic.

If you want to make bread using a pre-made packaged mix, you have a variety of options to choose ranging from quick breads to yeast breads.

Recommendation: Montina, a yeast bread mix made with Indian Ricegrass, is a powerhouse of fiber and somewhat resembles traditional wheat bread in terms of aroma and texture. Bob's Red Mill Natural Foods has a Hearty Whole Grain Bread Mix that captures the flavor of traditional rye bread with caraway seeds. For more brands, keep reading.

Option Four: Roll Up Your Sleeves.

Make your own bread from scratch using recipes found in gluten-free cookbooks.

Recommendation: Research and experiment with many different recipes from an array of cookbook authors. Be prepared to like many recipes, and dislike many too!

Option Five: Search-Engine It.

Type gluten-free bread into your favorite search engine and explore pages of options.

Recommendation: Choose wisely, but be willing to take a risk to find something you may love.

What are some brands of packaged gluten-free breads already sliced?

There is a limited selection of pre-made gluten-free breads. Keep in mind that most gluten-free breads that are packaged and sliced require refrigeration in the store and at home. Also, each company uses different flour blends in their recipes, so there is a variation in nutritional profiles of the breads as well as their texture and how well they hold together. While some breads will contain more white flours and starches to replicate traditional white bread, other companies will incorporate whole grain flours with color or more protein content that are naturally more nutrient-dense. Most pre-packaged and sliced breads found in the freezer section of your store will be more palatable after toasting. Many of the following brands can be ordered online also.

Ener-G Foods
 Varieties include Brown Rice, Tapioca, Egg-Free, Fruit, Hi-Fiber, Raisin, White Rice, Yeast-Free, White Rice Flax, Light White Rice, Four Flour, and Corn

Food For Life Baking Company
 Varieties include Raisin Pecan, Rice Almond, Rice Pecan, White Rice, Whole Grain Bhutanese Red Rice, Whole Grain Brown Rice, Whole Grain China Black Rice, Millet, Fruit & Seed Medley, and Multi Grain

Gillian's Foods
 Cinnamon Raisin, French, No Rye Rye, Sandwich, Sundried Tomato, and Roasted Garlic

Kinnikinnick Foods
 Varieties include White Sandwich Bread, Brown Sandwich

Bread, Italian White Tapioca Rice Bread, Raisin Tapioca Rice Bread, and Sunflower Flax Rice Bread

What are some brands of gluten-free bread mixes?

Nothing beats the aroma of a fresh hot loaf of bread baked in your home, even gluten-free bread. A variety of companies have patterned their signature style gluten-free breads after traditional favorite tastes, while other companies have no equal to their one-of-a-kind creations. Gluten-free bread mixes come in two recipe formats: quick bread or yeast bread. Quick breads are like cake batters made in loaf pans and are just that—quick—while yeast breads require time for rising and will often take a few hours to prepare. Either way, you'll eventually have a loaf you can slice, freeze, and enjoy.

Each bread mix utilizes different flours, some more nutritious and protein-rich than others. Some mixes are for making one type of bread only, while others can make different styles of bread using different company recommended recipes. Each bread will have its own moisture quality and flavor profile. Experiment to find the mixes you like best.

This list, which is by no means exhaustive, should help get you started stocking your new gluten-free kitchen with options for gluten-free bread. While some mixes are readily available in stores, some can only be purchased online.

Amazing Grains
Use Montina All-Purpose Flour Blend to make signature Montina Bread
Authentic Foods
All-Purpose Bread Mix and Cinnamon Bread Mix
Bob's Red Mill Natural Foods
Cinnamon Raisin Bread Mix, Cornbread Mix, Biscuit & Baking

Mix, Homemade Wonderful Bread Mix, and Hearty Whole Grain Bread Mix

Breads From Anna (Gluten Evolution, Inc.)
Gluten-Free Bread Mix, Banana Bread Mix, and Pumpkin Bread Mix

Gluten-Free Pantry
Favorite Sandwich Bread Mix, Yankee Cornbread, French Bread & Pizza Mix, Rye-Style Bread, Multi-Grain Bread, and Whole Grain Bread Mix

Miss Roben's
Noah's Bread Mix, White Sandwich Bread Mix, and Potato Bread Mix

Namaste
Bread Mix

Pamela's Products
Amazing Wheat-Free Bread Mix

Sylvan Border Farm
White Bread Mix, Classic Dark Bread Mix, and Non-Dairy Bread Mix

What are some brands of gluten-free pasta and noodles?

Thankfully, living gluten-free does not mean living pasta-free. But not all gluten-free pastas are created equal. The art of making gluten-free pasta is different from traditional pasta, and until fairly recently, gluten-free pasta had a reputation for falling apart or becoming mushy after cooking. But a variety of gluten-free pasta entrepreneurs have cracked the code secrets to making pastas that can please the most finicky pasta lover with mild, nutty flavors and great texture.

There are a variety of gluten-free pastas that use different flours in their formulations. Each has a unique taste, texture, cooking time, and performance quality. You'll be able to replicate many of your traditional pasta recipes using these varieties, many of which are made in the Italian tradition. Keep in mind that while some companies are specialty gluten-free companies by design, others have a gluten-free pasta product in their line but are not a 100 percent gluten-free facility. You'll want to make sure you are buying from a gluten-free company, or a company whom you've called to verify their manufacturing procedures and to confirm that their standards are suitable for your needs.

Ancient Harvest Quinoa Corporation
Shapes: Elbow, linguine, pagodas, rotelle, shells, and spaghetti
Flours used: Quinoa flour and corn flour

Annie Chun's, Inc.
Shape: Rice noodles
Flour Used: Rice flour

Bionaturae
Shapes: Elbow, fusilli, penne, and spaghetti
Flours used: Rice flour, potato flour, and soy flour

Eden Foods, Inc.
Shape: Soba noodles (Japanese)
Flour used: Buckwheat flour (Wheat-Free)

Heartland's Finest
Shapes: Elbow, lasagna, rotini, spaghetti, and ziti
Flours used: Whole navy bean flour and yellow corn flour

Orgran
Shapes: Corkscrew, lasagna, macaroni, penne, spaghetti, spirals, and tortelli, plus herb and animals
Flours used: Rice flour, corn flour, and millet flour

Papadini (Adrienne's Gourmet Foods)
Shapes: Linguini, orzo, penne, rotini, shells, and spaghetti
Flour used: Lentil bean flour

Thai Kitchen
> Shapes: Thin rice noodles and stir-fry noodles
> Flour used: Rice flour

Tinkyada Pasta Joy (Food Directions, Inc.)
> Shapes: Over 18 Italian-style pastas
> Flours used: Brown rice flour, white rice flour, and rice bran

What are some brands of gluten-free all-purpose flour blends for wheat flour substitution?

Having an all-purpose flour blend can be helpful when you're making gluten-free baked goods from scratch or when you're converting recipes to gluten-free versions. Many gluten-free all-purpose flours claim their product is a straight cup for cup substitute for wheat flour. Each blend will utilize different flours, have different nutritional profiles, and provide different baking performance characteristics. Many of the products have recipe suggestions or substitution tips on the package, and the company's Web site will often have recipes available for reference also.

Amazing Grains Grower Cooperative
> Product Name: Montina All-Purpose Flour Blend
> Montina (Indian Ricegrass), white rice flour, and tapioca flour

Authentic Foods:
> Product Name: Multi-Blend Gluten-Free Flour

Gluten-Free Pantry
> Beth's All-Purpose GF Baking Flour

Bob's Red Mill Natural Foods
> Product Name: Gluten-Free All Purpose Baking Flour
> Garbanzo bean flour, potato starch, tapioca flour, sorghum flour, and fava flour

Gifts of Nature
> Product Name: All Purpose Flour Blend

Brown rice flour, potato starch flour, white rice flour, chick pea flour, sweet rice flour, and tapioca flour

Mona's Gluten-Free

Product Name: Multi Mix

Organic brown rice flour, white rice flour, potato starch, tapioca starch, sorghum flour

Orgran

Product Name: Plain All Purpose Flour

Sylvan Border Farm

Product Name: General Purpose Flour

Potato starch, white rice flour, brown rice flour, amaranth flour, quinoa flour, white cornmeal, garbanzo flour, and soy flour.

Tom Sawyer Gluten-Free Products

Product Name: All-Purpose Gluten-Free Flour

White rice, sweet rice, and tapioca flours

What are some brands of gluten-free baking mixes?

A wide variety of gluten-free baking mixes feature different flours and other ingredients. Many are designed to create just one type of baked good, such as breads, brownies, cookies, cake or pie crust. But other mixes are designed to create a number of products using the same mix, such as muffins, scones, pancakes, and waffles. The recipes will have different names and instructions, but they will all use the same baking mix. Following is a list of some excellent versatile baking mixes.

1-2-3 Gluten-Free, Inc.

Aaron's Favorite Rolls, Allie's Awesome Buckwheat Pancakes, and more

Arrowhead Mills

Gluten-Free All Purpose Baking Mix (different from a flour blend), Wild Rice Pancake and Waffle Mix, Chocolate Chip Cookies, Vanilla Cake Mix, and Pizza Crust Mix

Authentic Foods

Vanilla Cake Mix, Chocolate Cake Mix, Lemon Cake Mix, Blueberry Muffin Mix, Pie Crust Mix, Pancake & Baking Mix

Bob's Red Mill Natural Foods

Brownie Mix, Chocolate Cake Mix, Chocolate Chip Cookie Mix, Biscuit & Baking Mix

Breads from Anna

Variety of bread mixes, including pumpkin and banana bread and a pie crust mix

Chebe Bread

Mixes featuring manioc flour and manioc starch. Use to make bread, bread sticks, pizza dough, and buns using company recipes. Makes Brazilian cheese bread rolls.

Dowd & Rogers, Inc.

Three cake mixes featuring Italian chestnut flour in Dutch Chocolate, Lemon, and Dark Vanilla varieties

Gluten-Free Pantry

A wide variety of mixes to make muffins, scones, cookies, cakes, pancakes, and breads

Hol-Grain

Chocolate Chip Cookie Mix, Pancake & Waffle Mix, Chocolate Brownie Mix

Namaste Foods

Bread, cakes, cookies, brownies, muffins, pizza crust, and waffle & pancake mix.

Pamela's Products

Baking & Pancake Mix, Chocolate Brownie Mix, Chocolate Cake Mix, Chocolate Chunk Cookie, and Wheat-Free Bread Mix

Who supplies individual gluten-free flours and starches?

Say good-bye to wheat and say hello to so much more. There are a variety of companies that sell individual gluten-free flours and starches separately for your baking and cooking needs. Check packages for gluten-free designations and call manufacturers to inquire about gluten-free manufacturing and testing procedures if you do not see a gluten-free designation on the package.

Arrowhead Mills

Buckwheat flour, flaxseed meal, millet flour, soy flour, white rice flour, and yellow corn meal

Authentic Foods

Almond meal, arrowroot flour, brown rice flour superfine, Garfava flour, garbanzo flour, potato flour, potato starch, sorghum flour, sweet rice flour superfine, tapioca flour, white corn flour, and white rice flour superfine plus cornstarch

Bob's Red Mill Natural Foods

Almond meal/flour, amaranth flour, arrowroot starch, black bean flour, brown rice flour, buckwheat flour, coconut flour, cornstarch, fava bean flour, flaxseed meal, garbanzo bean flour, green pea flour, hazelnut meal/flour, millet flour, potato flour, potato starch, quinoa flour, rice bran, sweet white rice flour, sweet white sorghum flour, tapioca flour, teff flour, white bean flour, and white rice flour

Dowd & Rogers, Inc.

Italian chestnut flour imported from Italy

Ener-G Foods

Brown rice flour, tapioca flour, potato starch, sweet rice flour, and white rice flour

Heartland's Finest
   Navy bean flour and pinto bean flour
Hodgson Mill
   Brown rice flour, corn starch, and soy flour
Nu-World Amaranth
   Amaranth flour, toasted amaranth flour, and amaranth starch
Simply Coconut
   Coconut flour
The Ruby Range
   Teff flour and mesquite flour
The Teff Company
   Maskal teff flour

Who are some suppliers of gluten-free grains?

The gluten-free food movement is bringing many gluten-free grains into fashion—and one does not have to be gluten-intolerant to enjoy the culinary flavors, recipe versatility, and nutritional profiles of these staples. Therefore, if the entire household doesn't follow the gluten-free way, these grains can make a happy compromise for the whole family when prepared in gluten-free recipes.

Ancient Harvest
   Traditional quinoa and Inca Red quinoa
Arrowhead Mills
   Amaranth, buckwheat, hulled millet, and quinoa
Bob's Red Mill Natural Foods
   Amaranth, buckwheat, millet grits, hulled millet, quinoa, and teff
Lotus Foods
   Whole grain rice varieties including Bhutanese Red, Forbidden Rice, Jade Pearl, Kalijra, Carnaroli, and Jasmine

Lundberg Family Farms

Whole grain rice varieties including various versions of brown rice, white rice, gourmet rice, and blends

Nu-World Amaranth

Puffed amaranth and rolled flakes

The Birkett Mills

Pocono buckwheat groats and Kasha (roasted buckwheat groats)

The Teff Company

Maskal teff grain

White Mountain Farm

Organic black and tan quinoa

What are some brands of gluten-free cereal?

If you enjoy beginning your day with cereal, there are many options from which to choose, both cold and hot. You'll find cereals made from a wide spectrum of nutritious gluten-free grains and flours such as amaranth, buckwheat, millet, quinoa, brown rice, and bean flours. To broaden your options, remember also that you can take individually packaged, gluten-free grains and make delicious, hot cereals and porridges using recipes designed for those grains often provided by the manufacturer or found in a gluten-free cookbook. Remember: Call the manufacturer if you don't see a gluten-free designation on the package.

AltiPlano Gold

Features organic quinoa hot cereals

Ancient Harvest

Quinoa flakes

Bakery On Main

Apple Raisin Walnut Granola, Cranberry Orange Cashew Granola, Extreme Fruit & Nut Granola, Nutty Cranberry Maple Granola

Barbara's Bakery
Puffins (some varieties are wheat-free but not designated as gluten-free)

Barkat
Organic Porridge Flakes made from rice and millet

Bob's Red Mill Natural Foods
Mighty Tasty Hot Cereal, Creamy Brown Rice Farina, Roasted Kasha

Ener-G Foods
100 percent Rice Bran

Enjoy Life Foods
Cinnamon Crunch Granola, Cranapple Granola, Berry Granola, and Very Berry Crunch

Heartland's Finest
CereOs (Cinnamon, Original, and Raspberry) made with rice flour and pinto bean flour

Nature's Path
Organic Crispy Rice Cereal

Nu-World Foods
Original Snaps, Peach Os, and Puffed Cereals made with amaranth

Perky's Natural Foods
Apple Cinnamon and Original PerkyOs, Nutty Flax, Nutty Rice

The Birkett Mills
Cream of Buckwheat

What are some brands of gluten-free oats?

If you've done your research on the gluten-free oats debate (Chapter Three) and have decided to introduce gluten-free oats into your diet, the following four companies are good places to start. As this segment of the industry continues to grow, it's likely more companies will begin to specialize in gluten-free oats or introduce the product to their existing lines.

1. Bob's Red Mill Natural Foods
   www.bobsredmill.com
   800-349-2173
   Rolled Oats and Steel Cut Oats
2. Château Cream Hill Estates
   www.creamhillestates.com
   866-727-3628
   Lara's Whole Grain Oat Flour
   Lara's Oat Groats
   Lara's Rolled Oats
3. Gifts of Nature, Inc.
   www.giftsofnature.com
   888-275-0003
   Certified Gluten-Free Whole Groats
   Certified Gluten-Fee Rolled Oats
4. Gluten Free Oats
   www.glutenfreeoats.com
   307-754-2058
   Old Fashioned Rolled Oats

What are some brands of packaged, ready-to-eat cookies, biscotti, brownies, and other baked delights?

There are many gluten-free options for sweets that feature different flours, flavors, and recipes. While some delights come right out of the box, others can be conveniently baked one cookie at a time, or made-to-order with a phone call. The following list scratches the surface of what's available. Keep in mind that companies often add new products or discontinue some flavors—tracking what they offer can be a delicious endeavor in itself! Experiment and find those that suit your fancy most. Bottom line: With all the varieties available, there's no excuse for having unsatisfied cravings.

Arico Natural Foods

Cookies including Double Chocolate, Chocolate Chunk, Almond Cranberry, Triple Berry, Lemon Ginger, and Peanut Butter

Bête Noire Chocolates

Specialty, vegan, gum-free cookies, biscotti, and other baked delights made to order.

Celia's Gourmet

Crispy Thumbprint Cookies, Chocolate Chip Cookies, Biscotti, and Macaroons

Enjoy Life Foods

Chocolate Chip, Snickerdoodles, Gingerbread Spice, Happy Apple, Lively Lemon, and no-oats "oatmeal" cookie varieties and Double Chocolate Brownie

Glutenfreeda Foods, Inc.

Refrigerated cookie dough known as Real Cookies

Gluten Free Kneads

Frozen cookie dough balls in Old Fashioned Chocolate Chip, Chocolate Toffee Crunch, Peanutty Butter, Snickerdoodle, Triple Chocolate Blast, and Lemon varieties ready-to-bake

Glutino

Vanilla Dreams, Chocolate Dreams, Shortcake Rings, and Chocolate Cream Filled Wafers

Jennie's

Coconut macaroons

Josef's Gluten-Free

Sugar cookies, vanilla chocolate filled sandwich cookies, and graham crackers

Mariposa Baking Company

Brownie flavors include triple chocolate truffle, walnut truffle, and mocha truffle. Biscotti flavors include almond, anise, cinnamon toast, ginger spice, orange walnut, and rustic raisin;

biscotti crumbs; and gift sets.

Nana's Cookie Company

Singular cookie flavors include Chocolate, Chocolate Crunch, Lemon, and Ginger. Cookie bar flavors include Berry Vanilla, Chocolate Munch, and Banana

Pamela's Products

Butter Shortbread, Shortbread Swirl, Spicy Ginger, Double Chocolate, Lemon Shortbread, Peanut Butter, Chocolate Chip Walnut, and Chunky Chocolate; Biscotti

Whole Foods Market (Gluten-Free Bakehouse)

A wide variety of their own Gluten-Free Bakehouse brands including breads, muffins, biscuits, scones, cakes, cookies, and pies

What are some gluten-free snack bars and nutrition/energy bars?

Gluten-free snack bars are plentiful, and this list mentions just a sprinkling of them. Featuring a wide range of gluten-free whole grain ingredients, snacking has never been so nutritious. These bars will help satisfy cravings any time of day and are great for outdoor excursions and fitness activities. Those who don't live gluten-free can benefit from these nutritious bars also.

AllerEnergy

Snack bars made with crisp brown rice, puffed millet, amaranth, and other ingredients

Arico Natural Foods

Snack bars that feature organic brown rice whole grain flour, rice starch, rice protein, and other ingredients

BumbleBar Foods, Inc.

Organic snack bars featuring sesame and flax seeds

Glutino
   Breakfast bars featuring chickpea flour and other ingredients

Kind Fruit + Nut Bars
   Fruit and nut bars featuring different dried fruits, nuts, and coconut

Lärabar/Humm Foods, Inc.
   Nutrition/energy bars featuring dried fruits and nuts

Leda Nutrition
   Snack bars made with chickpea flour, corn flour, tapioca flour, and rice flour

Organic Food Bar
   Nutrition bars featuring phytonutrient-dense formulations with organic brown rice protein

Orgran
   Fruit filled bars featuring milled corn, milled chick pea, and tapioca

Oskri Organics
   Snack bars featuring sesame seeds

Pear Bars
   Fruit bars containing fruit puree, pieces, and concentrates

Pure Bar
   Snack bars based on the raw foods concept, featuring brown rice protein, agave nectar, cherries, cocoa, cinnamon, nuts, and dates

Spring Bakehouse
   Nutballz energy cookies featuring brown rice flour, pinto beans, peanut butter (or almond), and other ingredients

What are some brands of gluten-free frozen meals?

For those days when you'd simply like to pop dinner in the microwave and be done with it, there are some options for gluten-free frozen entrees. Most gluten-free frozen foods are available in natural foods stores, and you can find a few from online shopping malls. As the market for gluten-free foods continues to grow, this category will further develop and provide more options. And with the new labeling regulations currently in effect and on tap for the future, at least you will be able to scan many selections in freezer cases quickly to determine gluten-free status. Some natural, gluten-free options often found in natural food stores or online shopping venues include

Amy's Kitchen, Inc.
Select entrees designated as "No Gluten Ingredients" or "Gluten-Free"

Annie's Homegrown, Inc.
Vegetarian Indian entrees under the name Tamarind Tree

Dr. Praeger's
Potato Crusted Gluten-Free Fish Fillets and Fish Sticks

Ethnic Gourmet
Select entree products are gluten-free

Lean On Me
Varieties of quiche

Mimi's Gourmet
Chili

Nature's Hilights
Rice pizza and brown rice pizza crust

Tandoor Chef
Select entrée products are gluten-free

Van's International
Waffles

What are some brands of gluten-free crackers?

Reading the ingredient labels of gluten-free cracker packages is a crash course in learning the many different types of gluten-free flours used. Because crackers are so convenient, options to experiment are abundant. The majority of gluten-free snack-crackers are also nutritious and use only natural ingredients, many of which are organic and wholegrain, unlike many of the wheat-based crackers found in mainstream supermarket shelves, which contain preservatives and fillers. Gluten-free crackers give you another avenue to healthy snacking habits.

Blue Diamond
   Nut Thins in almond, hazelnut, and pecan varieties
Edward & Sons Trading Company
   Brown Rice Snaps featuring organic brown rice flour in onion, plain, onion & garlic, and vegetable varieties
Ener-G Foods
   Cinnamon Crackers and Seattle Crackers featuring corn flour, corn starch, soy flour, and potato flour
Glutano
   Cracker Breads, Soda Crackers, Crispbreads, Wafers, Tea Biscuits, and Sesame Crackers featuring rice flour, corn or potato starch, bean flour, and ground rice
Health Valley
   Rice Bran Graham Crackers featuring organic brown rice flour, organic corn flour, organic soy flour, and rice bran
Lundberg Family Farms
   A variety of rice cakes featuring organic California grown rice
Mary's Gone Crackers
   Featuring organic brown rice, flax, sesame seeds, and quinoa in black pepper, caraway, herb, onion, and original
Miss Roben's
   Mock Graham Cracker mix featuring brown rice flour, white rice flour, and potato starch
Nu-World Amaranth
   Amaranth Mini-Ridge Crackers in Sun-Dried Tomato Basil

flavor featuring amaranth flour and yellow pea bran
Orgran
A variety of Crispbreads featuring corn and rice
Real Foods
Corn Thins featuring corn, brown rice, millet, sorghum, and buckwheat

What are some brands of gluten-free potato chips?

When you discover that certain packages of potato chips contain wheat or can't be eaten because of cross-contamination issues at the manufacturing facility, you may not only be surprised, you may fear that you won't be able to enjoy this favorite snack food again. But for gluten-intolerant potato chip lovers, there are options if you're willing to search for them. Read labels carefully to ensure the product is gluten-free and meets your approval from a gluten-free manufacturing perspective. You may have to call the manufacturer to inquire. And remember that one or more "flavors" in a company's product may be gluten-free, while others may not be. Those with barbeque seasoning and other flavors, for example, are immediate suspects for gluten.

There are many gluten-free potato chips that are privately labeled for individual stores. Below is a sampling of brands that have gluten-free potato chips:

FritoLay
Their website posts a list of their products that do not contain gluten.
Pinnacle Gold
Original Potato Chips
The Cape Cod Potato Chip Company
All flavors except Beachside Barbeque

What are some brands of gluten-free soy sauce and other sauces?

You can transform a multitude of Asian recipes into gluten-free celebrations if you have a wheat-free, gluten-free sauce! Thankfully, you have some options.

Mr. Spice
Garlic Steak Sauce, Ginger Stir Fry, Honey BBQ, Honey Mustard Sauce, Hot Wing Sauce, Indian Curry Sauce, and Thai Peanut Sauce

Premier Japan (Edward and Sons Trading Company)
Organic Teriyaki Sauce

San-J
Organic Reduced Wheat-Free tamari Soy Sauce

Sanchi
Organic tamari Soy Sauce

Other Asian and American sauces known for hidden gluten are becoming easier to replace as manufacturers formulate the traditional sauces without the wheat. Below are a few brands to explore:

Annie's Naturals
Organic BBQ Sauce Original

Daddy Sam's
Bar-B-Que "Sawce," Ginger Jalapeno Bar-B-Que "Sawce," and Salmon Glaze

Thai Kitchen
Spicy Tai Chili, Sweet Red Chili, Plum Sauce, Fish Sauce, and Peanut Satay

The Wizard's—Edward and Sons Trading Company
Wheat-Free Vegetarian Worcestershire

What are some brands of gluten-free beer?

Several foresighted entrepreneurs have taken the "gluten-free challenge" straight to the hops tank and have found means to brew a gluten-free beer. Using alternative gluten-free grains like sorghum and buckwheat, the methods of crafting traditional beer are being harnessed to produce gluten-free beers, ales, lagers, stouts, and more.

While the majority of gluten-free beers come from small, microbrew operations with limited availability, Anheuser-Busch was the first mainstream beer giant to break into the market with their version of gluten-free beer. Gluten-free beer availability is still spotty and finding it can be challenging, but patience will be rewarded over time as the market develops. Look for gluten-free beer locally in grocery markets that cater to the natural food consumer, liquor stores, and inquire at restaurants. And when traveling in Europe, you may find your options are even more abundant. Ask your neighborhood liquor store to order the gluten-free beer brand you favor if they don't carry it.

Anheuser-Busch
    Product Name: Redbridge
Bard's Tale Beer Company
    Product Name: Bard's Tale Dragon's Gold
Lakefront Brewery, Inc.
    Product Name: New Grist
Ramapo Valley Brewery
    Product Names: HB Honey Kosher Beer and Skull Crusher

What about soy milk and rice milk?

Always read the labels for gluten-free designation on these beverage products, and consider checking with the manufacturer if you are unsure. The manufacturing process of these beverages may include barley protein enzymes—which contain gluten—but you won't usually know because the ingredient list generally doesn't include these enzymes. Even though this kind of beverage may appear to be gluten-free on the package, the process by which it's made can turn the tables on you. However, the residual gluten left behind by the enzymes after manufacturing may test at a low enough level that is suitable for you. Check with your physician on which dairy-free beverages will be suitable for your diet. Silk Soymilk and Taste the Dream offer gluten-free soy and rice beverages.

What are some companies that have 100 percent dedicated gluten-free facilities or dedicated equipment for certain gluten-free products?

Below is a partial listing of food manufacturers mentioned in this book that make gluten-free food products in either a 100 percent dedicated gluten-free facility or have designated equipment or space for manufacturing a particular gluten-free product. Remember: When a company does not have a dedicated facility, always double check with the manufacturer for an explanation of their practices. Ask if they test their products for gluten and what the results are.

1-2-3 Gluten-Free, Inc.
Amazing Grains Grower Cooperative (Montina)
Ancient Harvest Quinoa
Annie's Homegrown, Inc.
Authentic Foods
Aunt Candice Foods
Bob's Red Mill Natural Foods
Breads from Anna
BumbleBar Foods, Inc.
Celia's Gourmet

Edward and Sons (Rice Snaps)
Ener-G Foods
Enjoy Life
Food Directions, Inc. (Tinkyada Pasta Joy)
Gifts of Nature
Gillian's Foods, Inc.
Gluten Free Kneads
Gluten-Free Pantry/Glutino
Glutenfreeda Foods, Inc.
Heartland's Finest
Lärabar
Leda Nutrition
Mariposa Baking
Mary's Gone Crackers
Miss Roben's
Mona's Gluten-Free
Nature's Hilights, Inc.
Namaste Foods
Nu-World Amaranth
Pamela's Products
Prima Provisions Co. (Chebe Bread)
Sylvan Border Farm
The Birkett Mills
The Really Great Food Company
The Teff Company
Whole Foods Market Gluten-Free Bakehouse

Chapter 7

STAPLE INGREDIENTS: BROADENING YOUR PANTRY

- What is amaranth?
- What is buckwheat?
- What is Indian ricegrass/Montina?
- What are Job's tears?
- What is millet?
- What is quinoa?
- What is ragi?
- What is sorghum?
- What is teff?
- What is the difference between brown rice flour, white rice flour, and sweet white rice flour?
- What is the difference between potato flour and potato starch?
- Is there a difference between tapioca flour and tapioca starch?
- What is xanthan gum?
- What is guar gum?

What is amaranth?

Today, along with other nutritious gluten-free grains like quinoa and teff, amaranth is enjoying a renaissance as a whole grain used in cooking, as well as a flour in gluten-free baking. Amaranth is a seed crop native to South America and was the essential food staple of the ancient Aztecs and Incas. This tiny seed is a nutritional powerhouse that contains each of the essential amino acids, in addition to boasting 6 grams of protein and 6 grams of dietary fiber in just one ½ cup serving. Similar to quinoa, this South American supergrain lends itself well to culinary versatility. Amaranth can be used in a variety of ways, ranging from porridge and pilafs to casseroles and snacks. Consider taking some of your favorite rice, potato and pasta dishes and substituting amaranth for a new taste and texture sensation.

These tiny seeds remain miniscule even after cooking, but become soft and tender while maintaining a faint, appealing crunch. Amaranth does not fluff up like rice and quinoa when cooked, but maintains a hearty, dense quality that maintains moisture well and has a unique, golden shimmer.

It's common to see amaranth flour being incorporated into flour blends for gluten-free baking; the high protein content provides a stickiness that is beneficial. But amaranth is also widely used in commercial food products. For example, NuWorld Amaranth specializes in a variety of ready-to-eat amaranth foods.

What is buckwheat?

It's easy to immediately assume that buckwheat is a grain that contains gluten because of the "wheat" in its name, but buckwheat is gluten-free and in fact has nothing to do with the wheat family. Indigenous to Russia, buckwheat is not a cereal grain as one might suspect, but rather an herb plant with edible, triangular seeds. The flavor of buckwheat is robust and people tend to either love it or hate it from first taste.

Buckwheat comes in the form of groats or kernels that can be used creatively in a variety of recipes ranging from soups and casseroles to desserts and entrees. Groats come in fine, medium, and course versions. Mild in flavor, groats cook particularly fast and have a unique texture that is unlike other gluten-free grains; softly tender with just a hint of crunch, buckwheat groats cannot be compared to rice, quinoa, amaranth, or millet in terms of texture. For recipe ideas, visit The Birkett Mills at www.thebirkettmills.com.

Seek out recipes that feature buckwheat groats coupled with flavors and imaginative ingredients that complement their mild flavor. Consider cream of buckwheat for a nutritious breakfast porridge. Toasted buckwheat, known as Kasha, is a popular dish in Eastern Europe, and the famous Japanese Soba noodles are made with buckwheat—however, beware, because these noodles commonly contain wheat flour.

High in protein and lysine, buckwheat is a nutritious gluten-free option that features an array of vitamins, including B and E, as well as minerals. Buckwheat can be ground into flour, either dark or light, and has a hearty flavor that gives buckwheat pancakes their unique flavor and aroma. Buckwheat flour can be used as a complementary flour to your gluten-free flour blend to impart protein and a rich flavor to your gluten-free baked goods.

What is Indian ricegrass/Montina?

Indian ricegrass was once a food staple for Native Americans in the western region of the United States. Not related to rice, Indian ricegrass has the acronym IRG and is known in scientific terms as *Achnatherum hymenoides*. Valued by Native Americans for its drought resistance and nutritive properties, this resilient wild seed grass grew in dry and sandy soil in the prairies extending from Southern Manitoba, Canada, to the highlands of Southern California. Indian ricegrass has made a twenty-first-century agricultural comeback, sparked by the need to serve the growing gluten-free food industry with more flour options. Through years of extensive research and development, the grower collective of Amazing Grains based in Ronan, Montana, in connection with scientists at Montana State University, brought this old Native American staple to the marketplace.

Indian ricegrass has a hard seed coat and is planted in the fall. It usually takes one year to grow a large enough crop to yield a worthwhile harvest. The brownish green color of the grass is hearty and robust and its slightly woodsy scent brings flavor and aroma to gluten-free baking.

Indian ricegrass is the signature ingredient in all Montina products. It's high in protein and fiber and is combined with a proprietary blend of white rice flour and tapioca flour to create the company's All-Purpose Baking Flour Blend, which provides 7 grams of protein, 5 grams of dietary fiber, and 5 grams of insoluble fiber per 2/3 cup. The Montina Pure Baking Supplement (100 percent Indian ricegrass) provides 17 grams of protein, 24 grams of dietary fiber and 24 grams of insoluble fiber. Indian ricegrass as milled flour is a good option for helping to bring dietary fiber to the gluten-free diet in the form of a baking supplement. However, Indian ricegrass in its whole seed form is not edible.

What are Job's tears?

One of the beautiful aspects of gluten-free living is that it can broaden your culinary horizons with strong international influences. Job's tears are another naturally gluten-free grain that may enjoy a renaissance in North America as the gluten-free food movement continues to gain predominance. Known in Japan as *hato mugi* and as *yimi* in Chinese, this beautiful gluten-free grain resembles large pearls of barley in the shape of a tear drop. While barley is often used in soups and stews, you can substitute Job's tears and never feel slighted. Although not as common as the other gluten-free grains, Job's tears are a traditional Eastern grain and deserve a try at least once on your gluten-free journey. With their delightfully tender texture and flavor that exudes a hint of corn, Job's tears will bring a twist of taste to your gluten-free adventures at home. These gluten-free pearls become creamy when cooked.

Job's tears have a sound nutritional profile and make a nice addition to your gluten-free cupboard. You can find Job's tears in Asian markets, health food stores, and via mail-order. This charismatic import fetches a higher price, but you may find the experience well worth the cost. Job 's tears are not as readily available as other gluten-free grains and you should check with the manufacturer regarding their manufacturing process of this grain to ensure no cross-contamination with wheat.

What is millet?

Going on a gluten-free diet gives you the opportunity to explore ingredients you may never have otherwise discovered, and millet is one such ingredient. Millet is a food staple among populations in Asia and Africa, but is typically far off the radar of an American diet until becoming gluten-free brings it to your attention.

Often used in birdseed, millet is an ingredient that imparts nutritious properties and culinary versatility to gluten-free cuisine and baking. Bland in flavor and similar in appearance to corn meal, millet is well suited for adding sweet or savory flavors to a variety of dishes, including snacks. Millet is versatile in texture and can be fluffy for pilafs and moist and sticky for porridges and polenta. When used as flour, it adds texture and fiber to baked goods.

Millet comes in the following forms: hulled for cooking, grits/meal, flour, and even puffed for a unique cereal option. Millet is high in protein and features many nutrients including vitamin B, copper, iron, phosphorus, and manganese.

In her cookbook *Whole Grains Every Day Every Way*, Lorna Sass explores all of the gluten-free grains, but gives millet in particular some well-deserved attention. Sass' culinary flair makes this seemingly dull and flavorless ingredient take a commanding presence in an array of recipe suggestions, including using buttermilk and chives to create a savory alternative to mashed potatoes and coating puffed millet in chocolate for a sweet and crunchy delight.

What is quinoa?

Well loved for its nutrition, taste, texture, and culinary versatility, quinoa is a gem in the repertoire of gluten-free grains. A time-honored food staple of South America and an essential food of the ancient Incas, quinoa is packed with cultural significance and history.

Scientifically speaking, quinoa is a seed, but it's commonly referred to in the generic sense as a grain, even as a "supergrain" because of its extraordinary health-promoting properties. From a nutritional perspective, quinoa can be considered near perfection. Similar to amaranth, quinoa has a good amount of protein, packing 6 grams of protein per ¼ cup serving. Quinoa contains all eight amino acids, making it a complete protein.

These beautiful seeds, found in black, ivory, and red, expand to a volume four times their original size after cooking. Easy to cook and digest, quinoa will broaden your culinary horizons on a gluten-free diet. Its versatility will make your gluten-free food adventures exciting if you like its unique taste and texture. Often compared to

Couscous (gluten!), quinoa cooks up light and fluffy like rice and can be substituted for any number of dishes. From soups and salads to side dishes, casseroles, and main entrees, quinoa will provide you with an abundance of creative options. Experiment! Try substituting quinoa for bulgur wheat in tabbouleh recipes. Or use quinoa for savory pilafs.

Quinoa flour is becoming more widely used in gluten-free baked goods. Look for quinoa flour in prepared baked goods and try to incorporate quinoa flour in your baking at home. Not only is this flour a nutritious option, it has favorable baking properties when you are looking to help replicate the gluten-effect.

What is ragi?

Once again, a gluten-free diet has the power to bring international flavor, tradition, and culture into the North American gluten-free kitchen with ingredients that you may never have otherwise discovered. One of the lesser known gluten-free ingredients, ragi is a gluten-free cereal grass that is not regularly mentioned in the lineup of gluten-free grains that includes amaranth, buckwheat, millet, sorghum, quinoa, and teff. More commonly known as finger millet or African millet, ragi is a nutritious food staple that is native to Africa and has also been cultivated for centuries in India, dating as far back as 1000 BC. Its flavor has a slightly bitter tone but is pleasant to the palate, and while the texture can have a gritty quality, its fiber content is similar to flax meal and has a sticky, viscous quality that will bulk up your dish.

In Africa, ragi is used to make porridge to accompany other foods. Ragi flour is widely used in India to make the well-known bread or leavened pancakes known as *Dosa*, or the less-leavened version known as *Roti*. Ragi roti is a traditional breakfast food of India that is made using ragi flour, grated coconut, onions, and green chilis. This food is often modified to include various vegetables as a stuffing like carrots, peas, and cauliflower.

While ragi flour is common in other cultures, to procure some ragi flour for your gluten-free North American kitchen is more challenging. But if you're looking to broaden your pantry's gluten-free ingredient profile, you may find the time well spent. Begin shopping for ragi flour in specialty Asian markets, spend some time online shopping for it, and browse Indian cuisine cookbooks for recipes utilizing this unique ingredient. As the gluten-free food industry continues to grow, ragi just might be an ingredient to watch.

What is sorghum?

Not widely recognized in the United States, sorghum is the world's third largest grain crop. As a whole grain, sorghum is also known as *milo* or *kafir* and is a key ingredient in regions of India and Africa. Sorghum grains are small and bead-like with a beige color. Like millet, sorghum is bland and dry, but when cooked it's best paired with ingredients that have moisture—like tomatoes—or by adding flavorful oils. In the United States, sorghum is mostly known for its sweet taste when it's extracted from the stalk and made into syrup or sorghum molasses, but the gluten-free food movement is bringing this shy ingredient into fashion.

When gluten-free baking was in its infancy, flours and starches made from rice, tapioca flour, and potato starch were the pivotal ingredients. While rice flour, potato starch, and tapioca flour are still widely used in gluten-free baking, sorghum flour is capturing the spotlight as a primary ingredient due to its baking properties that resembles wheat flour. Known for its high protein and fiber content similar to that of whole wheat flour, sorghum flour helps replace the gluten with its own "stretchy" characteristics and binding abilities. When added to other foundational flours, sorghum flour helps create baking versatility—flour blends that utilize sorghum flour are trumping the traditional flour blends that first originated in the early days of gluten-free baking. Carol Fenster is a proponent of sorghum flour and uses it regularly in her baking with flour blends throughout her cookbooks. Fenster says that sorghum flour is one of her favorite flours to work with.

What is teff?

A cereal grain indigenous to northern Africa (and a time-honored staple in Ethiopia), teff (or tef) is the smallest grain in the world, measuring approximately $\frac{1}{32}$ inch in diameter. For such a small grain teff is a nutritional powerhouse, packing all 8 amino acids, 6 grams of protein and 6 grams of dietary fiber per ½ cup serving. Plus, it's a favorable source of calcium and iron.

Teff comes in a variety of colors including black, brown, red, white, and ivory. As individually interesting as teff is in size, its flavor and texture are also unique. It has a mild, nutty flavor and when cooked it absorbs fragrant spices beautifully and takes on a texture similar to mashed potatoes. It lends itself well to creating savory hot porridges, polentas, and stews varying from sweet to savory. Teff is also favored as a finely ground flour that can be a nutritious addition to gluten-free flour blends for baking, as well as enhancing mixes designed for pancakes and waffles with protein and fiber.

The gluten-free Ethiopian flat-bread Injera is made with teff flour and has a taste and smell reminiscent of sour dough bread. With its flat, very-thin, pancake-like characteristics, this bread is often used as a "plate" upon which to spread savory sauces, stews, or mashes of legumes, then rolled up or folded over and eaten.

Tip: When considering eating Injera at a restaurant, always ask if they included wheat flour in the recipe because it is sometimes used in the United States to make this bread.

Gluten Free Kneads, a frozen cookie dough and focaccia company based in Austin, Texas, features teff flour in conjunction with amaranth flour in its Smart Flour Blend.

What is the difference between brown rice flour, white rice flour, and sweet white rice flour?

You'll find that the rice flours are as common to gluten-free baking as wheat flour is to traditional baking. There are subtle differences between these three flours, primarily with respect to baking performance. From a dietary fiber and protein perspective they are similar to each other, except that brown rice flour has approximately forty fewer calories per serving than sweet white rice flour. All three rice flours are lower in protein than whole wheat flour and each have approximately three fewer grams of dietary fiber per serving.

After the hulls of rice kernels are removed through the milling process, you are left with the starchy content of the rice grain and much of the nutritional content of the hull is no longer there. Rice flour can have a faintly sandy feel, and less finely ground brown and white rice flours can be a tad gritty to the touch as well as the palate.

Brown Rice Flour versus White Rice Flour

Whereas white rice flour is stripped of nearly all its nutrients after milling, brown rice flour maintains a few more and is slightly more nutritious than white rice flour. Brown rice flour naturally has a light brownish hue, while white rice flour is just that: white. While both flours are often selected as the main flour in a flour blend, in terms of baking performance, brown rice flour is a tad higher in protein, which can subtly enhance the extendibility of gluten-free dough.

Sweet White Rice Flour

This flour is made from glutinous (gluten-free!), short grain white rice commonly referred to as "sticky rice" in Asian cuisine. Due to its stickiness, sweet white rice flour helps bind the other flours in a recipe together and brings extension and pliability to gluten-free batters. It's often used as a portion of a flour blend in baked goods that require structure, like breads, muffins, and pie crusts. Sweet white rice flour shares a similar protein content to brown rice flour.

What is the difference between potato flour and potato starch?

Interestingly, these two ingredients are often mistaken for each other, particularly by the gluten-free baking novice. But there are some key differences that make these two flours almost as different as day and night.

Potato flour is heavy and dense to the palate because it's made from the whole cooked potato; potato starch is lighter in weight, as it's made only from the starch. Potato starch is similar to corn starch and is often used interchangeably.

Both potato flour and potato starch are rarely used alone in baking—they are generally added to complement the flour blend of a particular recipe. While potato flour can impart a chewy and moist quality to a baked good, potato starch will help bring a lightness to the product.

Potato flour maintains many of its nutrients, including protein and dietary fiber. Potato flour is made by cooking whole potatoes, drying them, and turning them into a finely ground flour. But potato starch has no protein or dietary fiber to speak of. Potato starch is processed from just the starch of the potato and this portion of the potato is not nutrient rich. Consequently, potato flour has nearly three times as many calories per serving. Potato flour is a "food" flour, whereas potato starch is more of an "agent" used to achieve a particular effect, like airiness in baking or thickening for sauces. You don't run to potato starch for its nutritional value. However, both potato flour and potato starch can be used in lieu of wheat flour for thickening sauces, soups, and gravies.

Is there a difference between tapioca flour and tapioca starch?

No, there is no difference. The terms "flour" and "starch" are used interchangeably to describe tapioca, which is made from the South American tuber root known as manioc, cassava, or yucca. Tapioca is often used to create a flour-blend partnership with rice flour and potato flour, or as starch in baked goods—this ingredient is most prized for its ability to bring a light quality to baked goods. Tapioca becomes chewy when baked and browns beautifully for a crust, as evidenced in the savory, chewy cheese bread rolls of Brazil known as *Pao de quejo*.

This stark white, powdery South American staple is a caloric-carbohydrate, but has virtually no protein, dietary fiber, fat, sugar, cholesterol, or sodium.

What is xanthan gum?

If you have never heard of xanthan gum before (pronounced *zan-thun*), you're not alone. Most consumers don't learn about this ingredient until going on a gluten-free diet. But xanthan gum has long been used in the food manufacturing industry in products such as salad dressings, milk products, dry baking mixes, chewing gum, and much more. The increasing need for ingredients that can help replace the gluten effect of wheat has brought attention to xanthan gum, which is also high in fiber.

Scientifically speaking, xanthan gum is a fermented sugar derived from corn. The end product is an odorless, powder-like substance with an off-white color. Xanthan gum is not a finished food or an ingredient that you can eat alone, like sugar or a spice, nor is it used to add flavor or nutritive value to a product. Rather, xanthan gum is used to produce a desired effect in making a food. It helps ingredients like gluten-free flours bind together, and helps give structure to baked products without gluten. When the powder is moistened, it becomes clear, sticky, and viscous. For example, xanthan gum provides viscosity for products like salad dressings. And when xanthan gum powder is moistened in a gluten-free bread batter or cookie dough, it helps bind the flours and other ingredients together, producing a sticky, gluten-like quality that keeps your gluten-free baked goods from falling apart.

What is guar gum?

Guar gum (pronounced like *gwahr*) is similar to xanthan gum—it is not an ingredient you eat alone, but is used to help ingredients bind together, thicken, and stabilize, and to create structure. Made from the seed of a cluster plant grown in India and Pakistan, guar gum is commonly found in commercial food products such as ice cream, puddings, cream cheese, and sauces. Guar gum is a powder that looks, smells, and feels like xanthan gum but is used less frequently in gluten-free baked goods. It is common to find gluten-free cookbook authors combine xanthan gum with a guar gum in the same recipe to capitalize on the structure building properties of both.

Gaur gum packs 6 grams of dietary fiber per 1 tablespoon. If consumed in excess, it can produce a laxative effect and it is recommended that only small amounts be used in baking. Use only as directed in recipes.

Both xanthan gum and guar gum are relatively expensive ingredients but are highly concentrated, and a bag will last you a long time.

Chapter 8

GROCERY SHOPPING: BASICS, TIPS, AND STRATEGIES

- Which stores have the best selection of gluten-free products?
- Where are gluten-free products located in the store?
- What should you know about prepared foods in the deli section and salad bar?
- Is it safe to buy gluten-free flours, grains, and other products from bulk bins?
- Are gluten-free products more expensive?
- How can you make your shopping experience more efficient?
- What should you do if you live in a small town?
- How do you get a store to carry a product you like?
- What should you know about and look for when shopping online?
- Where can you shop online for gluten-free products?

Which stores have the best selection of gluten-free products?

Accessibility to gluten-free products made by gluten-free companies varies from city to city, region to region, and, naturally, from store to store. The ease in which you can find gluten-free products locally depends on the unique demographics of your city. But regardless of where you live, visualize an inverted pyramid and divide it into thirds. The top third of the pyramid consists of stores that cater to the consumer interested in natural living and special diets. The majority of gluten-free products on the market typically fall into this category, as they are made without unnatural ingredients such as preservatives, artificial flavorings, colorings, and hydrogenated oils. Large chains like Whole Foods and Trader Joe's have ample shelf space to carry a full array of gluten-free products, and their customer base supports the large variety and quantities stocked on the shelves. Smaller, independently owned and operated natural food stores can often carry only as many gluten-free products as their shelf space and customer base will support.

In the middle section of the pyramid are large commercial grocery chains such as Albertson's, Kroger, and Publix that specialize in carrying the national supermarket brands. The natural foods sections in these stores are typically small, carrying only a tiny selection of gluten-free products, if any at all. Wal-Mart claims to stock hundreds of gluten-free products, but the majority of these products are not from dedicated gluten-free companies.

At the bottom of the pyramid are the specialty food stores that carry high-priced gourmet products, big box discount stores, convenience stores, and gas stations. You will not successfully fulfill your shopping list or meet your traveling food needs at these stores.

Where are gluten-free products located in the store?

Placement of gluten-free products in a store depends on the individual store and its customers, but there are a few general rules that can help you navigate and establish realistic expectations. Because natural foods stores usually carry a range of gluten-free products, it is not uncommon to find a store that dedicates an entire aisle or section to showcasing the gluten-free brands they carry.

In most natural food stores, you will typically find they stock the gluten-free products they carry manufactured by dedicated gluten-free companies next to the category you are looking for. For example, if you are looking for gluten-free pasta, it will be next to the wheat pasta, and the same goes for soup, sauces, canned foods, etc. A similar formula applies to finding baking mixes, cereals, cookies, flours, grains and salad dressings. Gluten-free bread and prebaked products are usually found in the freezer section. Some fresh gluten-free bread, cookies or muffins from a local bakery may be found in the bakery aisle of a natural foods store. Of course, products that are naturally gluten-free like eggs, butter, milk, fruit, and fresh meat will be found in their general category. In mainstream grocery stores, gluten-free products are becoming easier to find and are sometimes interspersed throughout the store, but they are typically found together in a small dedicated shelf area of the store geared for special diet needs.

When looking for gluten-free products for the first time it can be challenging because you are multi-tasking. You're busy looking for the products, reading labels, and recognizing and discovering certain brands. But after you shop a few times you become more familiar with locating the products and how to find new ones, and the process moves more efficiently.

What should you know about prepared foods in the deli section and salad bar?

Delis, buffets, and salad bars are laden with mystery and risk if you're not extremely careful—you must become a gluten sleuth if you'd like to eat from these. Usually, prepared foods in the deli case are made from a variety of both fresh and processed ingredients, and you have to be on guard for every processed ingredient used. At first glance, you will be able to immediately eliminate foods you know to visibly have gluten such as pasta salads, fried chicken, and many desserts. But other items such as soups, meatloaf, potato salad, and gravies need further inquiry because the gluten is not visible. These foods are gluten-guilty until proven gluten-free.

While some deli cases will have ingredient cards displayed for each dish, it's more common that they don't and you will have to ask the clerk to show you the recipe or package for something you are interested in. Having them recite the ingredients from memory can be helpful, but contains an element of risk if they forget to mention an ingredient which could have gluten. Plus, you won't know how particular ingredients were manufactured and whether they are 100 percent safe. From an investigative perspective, delis can be high-maintenance for the gluten-sensitive, so it depends on your level of desire, time to investigate, and willingness to take risks.

Salad bars usually do not have ingredient cards. Avoid obvious gluten-culprits like croutons, and be leery of foods such as soups, salad dressings, sour cream, and puddings.

Tip: Keep in mind that delis, food bars, and salad bars are also fertile grounds for cross-contamination issues, like a customer or employee inadvertently placing the tongs used to pick up croutons into the lettuce bin. And don't overlook the dangers of eating samples from alluring tasting tables and booths strategically placed at the end of aisles to tease your palate. Many times the product boxes or jars are not visible and you will not be able to read the ingredients. You can't assume those fetching corn chips and salsa are both gluten-free!

Is it safe to buy flours, grains, and other products from bulk bins?

Even though buying products from bulk bins can have price advantages, for the gluten-sensitive shopper they can present a mine field of invisible cross-contamination mistakes. If you choose to buy in bulk, it's necessary to keep the following in mind:

- If you're looking to buy gluten-free flours and grains, take a close look at where their bins are located in relation to the bins containing gluten-based ingredients. If the rice flour is in proximity to the all-purpose white flour, you run a high risk of the scoop for the gluten-free rice flour being inadvertently used for the wheat flour and put back into the bin, leaving traces of gluten. Similar scenarios can happen with particles of a gluten-based grain getting mixed into a gluten-free grain and what appears to be a gluten-free trail mix or dried fruit. Your chances of cross-contamination decrease if the gluten-free bin is out of reach from bins with gluten-based foods, but the risk is still present. Be extremely careful!
- Grocery store staff is mindful of properly maintaining the bins, but mistakes—like a gluten-based flour being accidentally poured into a bin labeled gluten-free flour—can and do happen.
- Bulk bins are not always labeled with full ingredient disclosure lists. While many foods may look enticing, it's hard to be 100 percent sure of what you're getting.

Bottom Line: Bulk bins are mystery bins, and your safety net is not fully in place when visiting them. Either be extremely cautious and know the possible consequences or avoid them entirely!

Are gluten-free products more expensive?

The general answer is yes. Some reasons for higher prices include

- The gluten-free food industry is growing fast to serve the increasing demand for gluten-free products, but the consumer market for these foods and ingredients continues to be a smaller segment of the population—the volume sales are far below that of major supermarket brands. Stores have to charge more for these products to make them worth the shelf space.
- Gluten-free packaged, ready-to-eat foods are typically more expensive than their wheat-based counterparts because the individual ingredients used to make the product are more expensive for the manufacturer to purchase.
- Many gluten-free products are found in the health food category instead of their specific food category (like the soups or pastas). They are often made with all natural, preservative free, non-hydrogenated, even organic ingredients, which are higher priced products. These higher production costs are reflected in higher prices for the consumer. Xanthan gum, an ingredient that replaces the gluten in wheat, is widely used and is also expensive, adding to the higher costs for both consumer and manufacturer.
- Many gluten-free products are made by smaller companies that use artisan methods and top quality ingredients to produce their products in relatively small batches. Companies making all natural gluten-free cookies in small batches can't offer the per cookie price that Nabisco does with its Chips Ahoy, for instance, packing dozens of cookies into each package.

- Artisan flours, starches, grains, and baking aids are produced in smaller quantities than wheat flour, and are subsequently more expensive.
- The economics of supply and demand is not bringing prices of gluten-free products down significantly—not yet. But in the meantime, celiacs with the proper paperwork from their doctor can write gluten-free foods off their taxes. It may not account for much, but you may be able to claim the differential of what normal foods on your shopping list costs versus the gluten-free versions. Consult with your tax advisor to learn more about how the IRS will allow an annual deduction. If this is for you, save those receipts!

How can you make your shopping experience more efficient?

When first learning how to shop gluten-free, the unfamiliarity of it all may seem tedious and frustrating. But don't worry—it gets easier and easier as you learn the ropes. Some steps you can take to help navigate your way through the store and make your experience less time-consuming and more efficient include

- Try to visit natural food stores because they specialize in carrying gluten-free products; your options will be more plentiful and members of the staff are often knowledgeable about these products. Many stores, like Whole Foods Market, offer regular gluten-free store tours.
- Ask the store manager if they have a typed list of the gluten-free products they carry. This tool is handy for finding them in the store and for making future shopping lists, to have for reference, and menu planning. Large national grocery chains typically don't have these pre-printed lists, but as with so many other

benefits that are coming to light with the growing awareness of the gluten-free diet, many stores are beginning to offer them.

- Research gluten-free manufacturer products before hitting the store by visiting Internet malls that cater to the gluten-intolerant consumers. You can scope out the offerings and make notes of the products and product manufacturers you would like to try, then see if your neighborhood grocer carries them. To get started, visit www.glutenfreemall.com or www.allergygrocers.com.
- Take your shopping list of staples that you usually buy and write down their gluten-free counterparts. For example, you can no longer buy American Beauty pasta, but you can find brands like Tinkyada Pasta Joy, Heartland's Finest, or Orgran. Online research ahead of time can help also.
- Never put anything in the cart without reading the label thoroughly. You don't want to get home only to find that your chicken broth contains wheat starch and have to return it.

What should you do if you live in a small town?

Shopping for gluten-free products is typically easier in metropolitan cities, because there are more stores that serve a larger population with a demand for gluten-free products—it warrants the supply. Living in a small town can be challenging particularly if you don't have a natural food store available. Plus, gluten-free products can be considerably more expensive to buy for both the shop owner and the consumer due to low-volume buying and higher transportation costs.

If you live in a small town, your approach to stocking your kitchen with gluten-free products will have a different strategy. Some options or guidelines to living gluten-free include

- Drive to the nearest big city where gluten-free products are widely sold, if the mileage makes it worth your while. Stock up on essentials each time you go.
- Ask your neighborhood store to carry or special order certain products for you. They may be happy to do this knowing that they will be immediately purchased by you, but expect to pay more than you would in a larger town.
- Consider shopping for a variety of products from online sources. You will need to increase your shopping budget to include shipping and handling charges, but the upside is that you can save money on sales tax through Internet shopping in most states.
- Buy larger quantities of the ingredients and products you go through quickly to cut back on trips into the city or to save on shipping and handling charges.
- Rely less on packaged ready-to-eat products and have quarterly gluten-free baking parties to make a variety of baked goods from scratch including cookies, muffins, and breads, then freeze them for future use. Make enough to last you for several weeks and have another party when you get low.

How can you get a store to carry a gluten-free product you like?

Not many consumers are aware of the power they can have to get products onto the supermarket shelves by simply letting the store know what you would like them to buy.

With small independently owned stores, it is easier to succeed because of the one on one relationship you can establish. Plus, you can bring certain products to their attention that they may not yet be familiar with.

But regardless of the size of the store, give it a try—many products have been placed on shelves through persistent demand from customers. Let them know that you will buy the product regularly if they make it available. Contact your local celiac community support group to let them know about the product, and that you plan to contact the local store to see if they would consider carrying it. See if any of the members would also like to voice their approval and support of the store carrying the product. Ask the group if they would consider mentioning the product and where it would be sold in their chapter newsletter. Take this information to the store and it will make your case even more appealing.

Or consider contacting the gluten-free product manufacturer directly. Provide them with the contact information of the store where you would like to have their product carried. They can call and try for the sale.

Keep in mind there may be a variety of reasons why a store won't carry a product. They may feel the retail price is too high for their customers, they can't buy it in volume, or they have a strict policy of buying through distributors. But go for it anyway!

What should you know about and look for when shopping online?

Many gluten-free brands can be purchased online, but many can also be found at your local supermarket or natural foods store—consider avoiding shipping and handling charges by seeing if your store carries the product first.

To find gluten-free foods on the Internet, enter specific words into your favorite search engine. The results can keep you busy for hours. Try search terms such as gluten-free foods, gluten-free products, gluten-free cooking, gluten-free recipes, gluten-free companies, or gluten-free shopping, or type gluten-free in front of the product you are looking for—such as gluten-free bread, gluten-free brownies, and gluten-free pasta.

Online shopping is particularly a boon for those who live in small towns and areas where gluten-free products are not readily available. In some cases, online resources are the only way gluten-sensitive individuals can purchase their foods.

However, unless you are shopping online from a respected gluten-free product manufacturer or an Internet shopping mall dedicated exclusively to the sale of gluten-free products, you need to be on guard and do your investigative work. You need to learn of all of the ingredients in a product you are considering and if they are not available on the Web site, call the manufacturer directly. While you are asking about the ingredients don't forget to ask if it is produced in a gluten-free environment, or how many ppms of gluten the product contains.

Where can you shop online for gluten-free foods?

Online shopping can be a godsend with respect to accessibility, but can be a hit to the pocketbook. And even though you may have access to a variety of natural foods stores in your hometown, online shopping malls open the door much wider to your options because of many factors, including shelf space, regional distribution, and local market demand.

You can often purchase gluten-free products directly from a company by visiting their Web site. Or there are a variety of gluten-free focused online shopping venues. And they usually provide foods that meet other dietary restrictions.

Keep in mind that online venues are like stores in that not all venues will carry the same products and prices may vary for the same exact product from mall to mall. Price shopping is alive and well in this market also!

Typically, gluten-free foods will be organized by category, such as pastas, breads, frozen foods, etc. Shopping online for your gluten-free foods can be hit or miss, particularly if you're shopping without product recommendations. But be willing to take risks to find those that you will buy again; all gluten-free products vary in terms of nutrition, texture, taste, quality, and price, so experiment to find the products that best suit you.

Tip: Consider buying in bulk when you can to avoid repeat shipping charges for repeat orders. Many gluten-free products freeze well, so you needn't worry about wasting food.

Currently, the largest gluten-free online shopping malls include

www.allergygrocers.com
www.celiac.com
www.glutenfree.com
www.glutenfreemall.com
www.glutensolutions.com

Warning: There are some food Web sites that have categories for "gluten-free foods." However, the products posted in those categories are not always gluten-free! Whether it's a sales trap or an unintentional mistake, always read the ingredients before making a purchase online.

Chapter 9

THE BATHROOM AND MEDICINE CABINET: LOOKING BEYOND THE KITCHEN

- Should you be concerned about gluten in personal care (topical) products?
- Is toothpaste gluten-free?
- Are your medications gluten-free?
- How do you read medication labels and inserts for gluten?
- Where can you find help researching the gluten-free status of medications?
- What are gluten-free alternatives to over-the-counter medications?
- Could your lipstick be making you sick?
- Are your nutritional supplements gluten-free?

Should you be concerned about gluten in personal care (topical) products?

Gluten-free personal care products deserve your attention and concern, as well as a conclusive set of guidelines for the gluten-free community at large to follow. Currently, there is no one definitive answer or set of rules regarding the use of topical products containing gluten, and when you ask this question, you will typically get two different answers.

One camp will say that in order for gluten to cause a problem for those with celiac disease, it must be present in the digestive tract—therefore, using topical products containing gluten will probably not be problematic unless you have dermatitis herpetiformis. However, the other camp says that anything you put on your body is absorbed and enters the blood stream. If you are intolerant to gluten, this absorption factor can be problematic and you should avoid gluten in personal care products.

It's important to do your research as well as consult your physician for guidelines on using topical products that contain gluten, but even if you've been given the green light by your doctor, it's still recommended to proceed with caution and monitor your reactions to the products you choose to use. Wheat-protein, for example, is commonly used in products such as soaps, bath gels, shampoos, conditioners, mascara, cosmetics, and moisturizers. The wheat-protein may not affect the intestine directly, but may produce symptoms in those who are highly sensitive, particularly if the case is dermatitis herpetiformis.

Bottom line: Those who react negatively to digesting gluten can also be sensitive to gluten when applied to and absorbed in the body via topical products. Exercise caution and decide for yourself what works and doesn't work for you topically. And if you've been following a gluten-free diet and feel great, but feel lousy after using a topical product containing gluten, it's possible you're reacting to the gluten or something else in the product and should discontinue use.

Is toothpaste gluten-free?

The majority of toothpastes are gluten-free, but take some time to check with the manufacturer of your favorite brand to confirm gluten-free status. For example, Colgate, Crest, and Tom's of Maine are just to name a few companies that have gluten-free toothpaste.

Are your medications gluten-free?

If you thought reading food labels for gluten-free status was challenging, get ready to take your label reading skills up a few notches and investigate the bottles and boxes in your medicine cabinet. As with many food products, medications are also gluten-guilty until proven gluten-free. To determine whether or not your medications contain gluten requires time-consuming research. Keep in mind that over-the-counter and prescription medications do not abide by the same labeling protocol as foods do, so knowing what to look for and reading very carefully are even more important with medications than food. Never assume a medicine is gluten-free, particularly if you can't read the cryptic language on the label. Medications can be havens for hidden gluten.

Making your medicine cabinet gluten-free deserves just as much vigilance as your kitchen: Remove everything from the cabinet, clean well, and let dry. Do not put anything back into the cabinet until you have determined its gluten-free status. You should even toss out your old toothbrush.

Sort your medications into two categories: those you take on a daily basis, and those you have on hand for occasional use. The ones you use daily will require immediate attention. But before spending time investigating the products you use infrequently, consider if you even want to bother. For example, instead of popping a throat lozenge or swallowing cough syrup, consider a gluten-free naturopathic remedy that can serve the same purpose, like gluten-free hot tea with honey and lemon or gargling with hot salt water.

Once you have sorted through what you need and want to keep, you're ready to start reading the labels and package inserts.

How do you read medication labels and inserts for gluten?

More drug manufacturers are beginning to remove allergens, including gluten, from their products, but this is an evolution in the industry and will take time. While companies reformulate their products to find other ingredients that will serve as binders, fillers, coatings, or diluents, you need to be very aware of any possible gluten.

You can begin by looking at the label on the package just to get an overview, but for thorough information it's best to go straight to the package insert for the ingredients. The first ingredient listed on the insert will be the chemical name of the product, and this is of no use to your investigation—look for the "inactive ingredients" list. In this section, you'll find words that will seem more familiar to you from reading food labels, and you have to determine the food source. For example, if you see words like starch, vegetable, malt, or protein, you need to take your investigation to the next level and call the product manufacturer. Any starch that is not identified with the food source, such as potato, rice, tapioca, or wheat, is automatically a suspect.

Also, if you find maltodextrin listed, beware. Even though this ingredient is usually gluten-free in foods in the United States, its status is unclear in pharmaceuticals, particularly if the drug was manufactured overseas.

Look for any ingredient that refers to "dusting powder." The source must be identified through the manufacturer.

And watch out for Dextimaltose, an ingredient that combines dextrin (gluten-free) and maltose (which can be produced from barley malt and makes this ingredient a suspect).

Where can you find help researching the gluten-free status of medications?

It's natural to think that your doctor should be able to tell you if the medications prescribed to you are gluten-free or not. But surprisingly, often the doctor will not know and will refer you to the pharmacist. And often, the pharmacist will not know and will refer you to the product manufacturer. As strange as this scenario may sound, when it comes to medications, you have to be the ultimate watchdog.

It's always best to start with the package insert and to thoroughly read through the language in the "inactive" ingredients section for words that raise red flags (i.e., an unidentified starch). But what happens if you don't have a package insert, or the slip distributed by the pharmacy was thrown away several doses ago?

The Physicians' Desk Reference (PDR) is an annually published guidebook that contains package insert information from the manufacturer on prescription drugs. The book is widely available in doctors' offices, libraries, bookstores, and can be purchased online. It's expensive, fetching $94.95 for the 2007 edition, so consider calling your local library first or ask if your doctor will allow you to glance at the office's copy.

You can also contact a national celiac disease support organization to ask for their recommendations on Web sites they trust with lists of drugs or helpful products for you to reference. But keep in mind the following about any Web site resource: they are often created and maintained by individuals like you and me, and their lists may not include all drugs, be fully updated, or be accurate. Ingredients can change without notice from a manufacturer. Always be cautious and use your discretion. When in doubt, call the drug manufacturer.

What are gluten-free alternatives to over-the-counter medications?

Researching medications and over-the-counter remedies to determine gluten-free status can be time-consuming and tedious. And naturally, you will have to undertake this task in varying degrees over the course of your gluten-free life. But going gluten-free gives you the opportunity to take an honest look at what you do take and question the true necessity of a product in your life, while being open to finding alternative approaches to feeling better.

It's of course recommended that you consult with your physician or nutritionist about treating ailments, but consider looking at the medications you keep on hand to treat fleeting conditions such as headache, heartburn, sore throat, congestion, constipation, diarrhea, itchy skin, and so forth, or pills created to do something such as control appetite, help you sleep better, energize you, enhance your sense of well-being and the like—could you remedy those situations with something other than medication?

Are you willing to forgo the hot and spicy food you know gives you indigestion so you don't feel the need to pop an antacid pill? To help constipation, can you pitch the laxative in favor of regularly incorporating more fiber and green leafy vegetables into your diet? What about exercising more to help curb your reliance on the sleeping aid? Not that the products you have chosen to purchase don't serve a purpose, but going gluten-free simply gives you a good excuse to think of your alternatives and perhaps saves you the time and energy of researching the gluten-free status of over-the-counter medications.

Could your lipstick be making you sick?

It seems ludicrous that gluten could have an effect on beauty and love, but the forbidden protein works in mysterious ways. Valued for its binding and strength-enhancing qualities, gluten is often used in cosmetics. Because lipstick is applied directly to the mouth it can be ingested via kissing, eating, and licking your lips. Therefore, lipstick must be on your radar too. Although transferred in relatively trace amounts and more so if several applications a day are the norm, the gluten found in your (or your wife or girlfriend's) lipstick may be just enough to be "poisonous."

If you wear lipstick, lip gloss, lip balms, or lip liner, it will behoove you to do your research on the brands you favor. Begin with the ingredient listing on the package to find any component that is wheat or gluten related. Wheat protein is a common ingredient in lip products. If you can't find any words on the list that suggest wheat, it's recommended that you still get in touch with the manufacturer to confirm. And keep in mind that if you confirm your favorite brand and shade is gluten-free, don't take it for granted. Manufacturers are known to change ingredients without notice. Look for alternative gluten-free brands and shades that could be suitable backups should your current gluten-free lipstick change ingredients, be out of stock, or get discontinued.

And what about kissing? Again, while trace amounts will only be ingested, it can be enough to cause concern. Who would have dreamt that kissing could be an area of concern on the gluten-free living radar?

Are your nutritional supplements gluten-free?

As with medications, manufacturers of vitamins and other nutritional supplements are not subject to the same labeling practices that food manufacturers must adhere to. However, many bottles and packages will include a list of allergens that are *not* present in the product. But always look for "gluten" to be listed. If the product simply lists that it contains no "wheat" or "barley," for example, that's not a clear enough answer for you. You need to see "gluten." Call the manufacturer to confirm.

Chapter 10

DINING OUT: SURVIVAL TACTICS AND PROACTIVE APPROACHES

- Are restaurants aware of the gluten-free diet?
- How do you begin reading menus for gluten-free foods you can and want to eat?
- What items on a menu should you be suspicious of?
- What are some risk factors in dining out?
- What can you do to help ensure a safe experience?
- What are some traditional gluten-free dessert recipes?
- What are the names of pasta shapes/noodles so you can avoid them?
- Will you need to educate your server or the chef about gluten-free ingredients?
- Can you trust a restaurant's gluten-free menu?
- Are some restaurants easier to dine out at than others?
- Where can you find gluten-free friendly restaurants in your city?
- What is a recommended routine to follow when dining gluten-free?
- How can you encourage your favorite restaurant to offer gluten-free options?
- Can you eat gluten-free at fast-food restaurants?
- Are bakeries off limits?
- What about coffee shops?
- When should you leave a restaurant?

Are restaurants aware of the gluten-free diet?

Gluten-free diet awareness in restaurants is improving throughout the United States, but the level of awareness varies dramatically from restaurant to restaurant, city to city, and coast to coast. There are more restaurants in large metropolitan cities that are aware of the gluten-free diet and have experience in serving customers with special diet needs than there are in smaller cities. But regardless of the size of city you live in, you will have to search out the establishments that can cater to your gluten-free diet needs, and avoid those who can't.

A growing number of restaurants are now offering gluten-free menus upon request—more and more, eating establishments are analyzing their menu and designating items as "gluten-free." However, many more restaurants who are aware of the gluten-free diet do not offer a separate menu, because the relatively small demand does not warrant it; they choose to handle gluten-free requests individually upon request. And then, unfortunately, there are too many restaurants to count that have not yet caught the wave. But give them time. They will.

Expect to look at each restaurant individually and ask the same questions of each one. Realistic expectations are important; it's important that restaurants cater to a customer's dietary restrictions where they can, but you can't expect all restaurants to provide a wide variety of gluten-free options, just as you can't expect a high-end jewelry store to sell cheap watches. Finding restaurants that are gluten-free friendly becomes a shopping experience and can be quite rewarding, like finding a store that sells fashions to suit your personal style.

How do you begin reading a menu for gluten-free foods you can eat?

Much like mystery novels, restaurant menus can keep you guessing—you will encounter twists and turns until you crack the case and decide what's safe to order. But before taking on the challenge of eating at a restaurant that does not have a gluten-free menu, you need to know what gluten is and where it is found (Chapter Three) so you can successfully avoid it. While you can ask your server about what is gluten-free on the menu to save time, it's wise to get into the habit of analyzing the menu yourself so you can be sure.

Look first to eliminate the obvious glutens: sandwiches because of the bread, pizza because of the crust, fried foods because of the flour batter, and pasta dishes because of, well, the pasta. After reading several menus in this fashion, you will get a feel for a menu's gluten-free ratio, the approximate percentage of possible versus impossible foods. The higher the ratio in favor of the possible options, the easier time you will have. Soon, you'll develop a personal intuitive-percentage that determines whether you stay at a restaurant or move on.

After eliminating the obvious gluten culprits, look more closely at meals that could be gluten-free, like entrée salads or meats with a gluten-free starch like rice or potatoes. These are possible foods, but your research is not through—you must find out if there's gluten hidden within them.

What items on a menu should you be suspicious of?

Unlike the obvious glutens like bread and pasta, hidden glutens make up just a small portion of the meal, but can have just as dangerous an effect if you are not careful to recognize and eliminate them. Some small glutens are elemental to certain recipes or styles of food preparation and can't necessarily be removed. These can include breading on meats, flour for dusting meats and fish before sautéing, breadcrumbs for meatloaf, crusts used for desserts, flour to thicken soups, wheat starch in frozen French fries, and barely to add flavor and texture to soups and stews. And you should always be on the lookout for gluten in things used for dressing up a meal, like sauces (always watch for soy sauce!) for savory and sweet items, gravies, salad dressings, flavorings, spice mixes, and dairy products like sour cream and ice cream. You will never know about these ingredients unless you ask and have a server investigate the product label or the recipe.

Also, be leery of beverage menus. Gluten is in beer and can hide out in a variety of beverages ranging from coffee drinks and milk shakes to liquors and cordials.

After you gain practice in reading menus, you will learn how to recognize even the smallest, most hidden of glutens. But don't take your gluten investigative hat off and pocket the magnifying glass just yet ...

What are some risk factors in dining out?

You can do your investigative work thoroughly and find foods to choose from on the menu that appear perfectly safe, but can still encounter danger if you don't ask key questions and take certain steps. Cross-contact (also known cross-contamination—see Chapter Two for more information) in restaurants can spoil your carefully researched gluten-free meal. It is your responsibility to be aware of this possibility and do your best to ensure it doesn't happen.

When first learning how to dine gluten-free, you will mostly be concentrated on reading the menu correctly and thoroughly. But beyond the menu, you must also think about what goes on behind the scenes in a restaurant and how to avoid common mishaps from unaware staff. Consider the following examples:

Common Risk Factor #1

You order a salad and request no croutons, but your server mistakenly adds them, remembers at the last second, and picks them off, leaving behind a trail of nearly invisible crouton crumbs on your lettuce.

Common Risk Factor #2

You order a steak without seasoning, but your steak was inadvertently pan seared in a pan that was used previously to grill a piece of chicken dusted with flour.

Common Risk Factor #3

You are craving a fried food at a Chinese restaurant and ask for the sesame chicken to be floured with potato starch instead of wheat flour, but the cook fries your chicken in the same fryer where wheat-floured meats are fried.

The next step is to be proactive to ensure your safety . . .

What can you do to help ensure a safe experience?

As well as finding the foods on a menu that you can eat, there are other proactive steps you must take to make sure you are served a gluten-free meal.

- Let your server know that you are gluten-sensitive and need your meal to be prepared using equipment that is thoroughly cleaned and free of any residual gluten from previous meal preparation. When the service staff is aware of your needs, they can help take every step possible with the chef or cooks to protect you.
- When ordering something you know to be gluten-free, think ahead about its preparation. Naturally, you don't need to become a chef to do this, but just knowing enough about how foods might be prepared will help you ask the right questions. For example, ask about breading or dusting meats with flour before ordering.

- Always ask questions when necessary to clarify ingredients and preparation methods.
- Never assume a restaurant is familiar with cross-contact issues and knows how to protect your food appropriately.

Cardinal Rules: Try to have an idea how your food is prepared from start to finish and confirm that sterile equipment has been used. Never let your guard down. Ask the server to hold items like the bun and request anything suspicious on-the-side, like salad dressing.

Reality Check: Determining the gluten-free status of any food on a menu depends on your investigative skills and the questions you ask. Even though asking questions of the staff is part of the gluten-free dining routine, frankly speaking, there will be times when you are simply not in the mood for asking detailed questions because they can be tedious and tiresome or you just don't feel like it. In these cases, it's important to remember the possible consequences if you don't follow through with protocol.

What are some traditional gluten-free dessert recipes?

Unfortunately, when it comes to the vast majority of desserts, the wheat is king and finding recipes and menu items that don't include wheat can be challenging. The list below provides a quick reference of recipe titles or ideas that are naturally gluten-free desserts that don't require flour of any kind. These recipes can be found in cookbooks, online resources, magazines, and other sources.

Baked Apples
Bananas Foster
Castagnaccio (Italian Chestnut Flour Cake)
Crème Brulee
Chocolate Soufflé*

Chocolate Ganache
Chocolate Fondue*
Flan
Flourless Chocolate Cake*
Fudge
Fruit Compotes
Junket
Meringue Cookies
Macaroons
Mousse
Panna Cotta
Peanut Brittle
Rice Pudding
Tapioca Pudding

*Note: While these recipes can occasionally call for flour in small amounts, it's not typically the case. When dining out, ask the server or chef to confirm that no wheat flour has been used in their recipe.

What are the names of pasta shapes/noodles so you can avoid them?

Numerous Italian dishes will include the name of the pasta shape in the recipe title without making reference to it being pasta. If you know the basic Italian pasta varieties, it can help you more quickly eliminate unsafe foods from your menu choices. Following are many common pasta names. Why list so many? Even though you can bypass the pasta section of a menu, it's not uncommon for a pasta shape to show up in a soup, stew or other dish. Knowing these names will help you recognize dishes including pasta immediately that could otherwise trick you. This list will be helpful when visiting Italian restaurants at home as well as abroad.

Bavette

Cannelloni (Manicotti)

Capellini

Cavatappi

Dischi

Farfalle

Fettuccine

Fusilli

Gigli

Lasagna

Lumaconi

Malfattini

Occhi di Passero

Orsetti

Penne

Pipette Rigate (Elbow Macaroni)

Radiatore

Riccioli

Rigatoni

Spaghetti

Tagliolini

Tagliatelline

Ziti

Bucatini

Capelli d'angelo (Angel Hair)

Casarecce

Conchiglie (Shells)

Ditalini

Farfalline

Francesine

Gemelli

Grattugiata

Linguine

Mafalde

Midolline

Orecchiette

Pappardelle

Pipe

Piombi

Reginette

Rigati

Rotini

Stelline

Tagliatelle

Tortiglioni

Will you need to educate your server or the chef about gluten-free ingredients?

It's natural to have high expectations of the chefs, managers, and servers in the restaurant industry. These professionals take care of us when we are in their establishments, and we often expect them to know everything there is to know about food because it is their business. Yet, it is common to find gaps in knowledge about special diets, or in some cases, a complete breakdown in communication. As you embark upon the gluten-free lifestyle and learn more about the dietary requirements, so too are people in the restaurant industry— and it will take time for the them to reformat their service protocol to best accommodate their guests with special dietary needs. In the meantime, simply understand that you may have to explain your needs thoroughly and carefully when eating out.

Be prepared to talk about what gluten is and where it's found. You will occasionally find yourself talking about the hidden gluten in various ingredients while getting bewildered expressions from your server. Also, be prepared to answer questions from the server or chef about the diet and if certain ingredients are gluten-free or not.

To make your dining experience as hassle free and safe as possible, you need to know your ingredients and do your research ahead of time. This way, you can best navigate your way safely around menus without having to rely on the staff to do it all for you. Think of educating your server or chef as an opportunity to help other dining guests because the more they know now, the better they can serve others later as well as you on your next visit.

Can you trust a restaurant's gluten-free menu?

As you become more seasoned in the art of gluten-free dining, you will develop a level of trust with certain restaurants. If you like the food and feel fine afterward, chances are good you will want to return. But you'll find also that the level of gluten-free food knowledge will vary from restaurant to restaurant, and just because a restaurant offers a "gluten-free" menu or designates items on the menu as gluten-free does not mean you can let your guard down. You can trust, but do so with your eyes wide open.

Double check their knowledge of ingredients used on the menu against yours. If you suspect a menu item that is designated as gluten-free has chicken broth or a beef base as an ingredient, for example, it will not hurt to simply ask if the broth is freshly made or comes from a package or mix. If it is packaged, you can have them confirm its gluten-free status with the ingredient label.

Ask if the restaurant knows exactly how a "gluten-free" ingredient was manufactured. Have they double-checked their ice cream? You have to be the devil's advocate with restaurants. Also, ask how they avoid cross-contact. Offering gluten-free pasta to replace traditional pasta does not serve you well if it's boiled in the same water used for boiling wheat pasta. While you should be able to trust the staff, restaurant professionals can make assumptions and mistakes about gluten-free status.

While it's the restaurant's responsibility to confirm each ingredient before designating a gluten-free item, it's still your responsibility to hold the line and cross-reference their knowledge where you believe it's necessary to do so.

Are some restaurants easier to dine out at than others?

With so many different restaurant formats and styles of cuisine, the task of finding something gluten-free can seem daunting. But as with shopping for clothes—certain stores are easier to shop at because they offer the styles you like—certain restaurants and styles of cuisine will be more accommodating to you.

Before heading out on any dining adventure, it's best to do your research into options that will be safest for you. Restaurants that cater to customers interested in healthy foods will often service many special diet needs, including the gluten-free diet. Also, servers are often knowledgeable about the ingredients and can guide you in the appropriate direction.

While gluten is often abundant in upscale cuisine, fine dining restaurants can sometimes be easier to eat at because of the slower pace of service and the finer attention to detail. At these restaurants, fulfilling a gluten-free diet request can be something they enjoy the challenge of and perform with style and pleasure. Executive chefs can often prepare something special for you upon request; the personalized service might take a while longer than you're used to, but it will be worth the wait.

Restaurants with gluten-free menus are obvious choices for making the dining experience easier. The Outback, P.F. Chang's China Bistro, and Pei Wei Asian Diner have corporate-designed gluten-free menus available at all of their locations. Maggiano's Little Italy regularly accommodates gluten-free requests without a designated menu. Fast-food restaurants, diners, bars, and restaurants that have gluten-focused menus, like most Italian places, will typically be more difficult to dine at because of limited options or fast-paced service.

Simply keep in mind that some restaurants are in tune with the times, and others are not. Some will take the extra steps to ensure a safe and pleasant experience for you while others may not have the ability, knowledge or ample time to serve you appropriately. And remember: the more processed the food, the more challenging your dining experience may be. Restaurants that focus on fresher, simpler foods can yield more options.

Where can you find gluten-free friendly restaurants in your city?

Besides researching restaurants through your own trial and error, there are a variety of resources you can consult when trying to find gluten-free friendly restaurants in your city or the cities you travel to.

- Check with the local celiac and gluten-intolerance community support group in your area. There may be more than one chapter to contact and each will have members familiar with a variety of good dining options in the city. These recommended restaurants may be listed on the chapter's Web site, in a local dining guide compiled by the members, or featured in chapter newsletters, and you can always get them by word of mouth.

- You can also submit a posting to celiac@listserv.icors.org, which is basically an online bulletin board that reaches a gluten-intolerant community of a few thousand individuals nationwide. Write that you are looking for gluten-free friendly restaurants in the city of your choice and wait for replies from the community.

- There are also many good books available that can recommend gluten-free restaurants for wherever you may be. An excellent resource is Triumph Dining (order online at www.triumph-dining.com); it contains thousands of restaurants recommended by celiacs, hundreds of restaurants with gluten-free menus, and lists of what you can eat safely at regional and national chains.

- Large cities typically have a restaurant association consisting of thousands of member restaurants. These associations may have lists that specify restaurants that can handle gluten-free diet requests or offer specific menu items.

- Type in gluten-free restaurants and the city of your choice in your favorite search engine; you should get lots of results to explore. You can also call the editorial staff at the food section of your city newspaper or lifestyle magazine and ask for any recommendations. More and more media outlets are featuring gluten-free friendly establishments in their city.

What is a recommended routine to follow when dining gluten-free?

As you dine out more and more under the specific regulations of the diet, you will develop your own personalized routine with steps you feel to be the most important for you to follow according to your own situation. The following list of steps are suggestions that may be useful to you when beginning to navigate through the dining scene. At first you might use all the steps, then gradually eliminate some as you become more comfortable. Eventually, your routine will become second nature.

- Call restaurants ahead of time to ask if a gluten-free menu or specific gluten-free items are offered. This can often save you a trip.
- Know what foods contain gluten and how to find hidden gluten before reading a menu, or bring your "safe foods" lists with you. This will save time and often eliminate the gluten guessing game.
- In unfamiliar restaurants, particularly when traveling, scan the menu before sitting down to determine if the gluten-free ratio is acceptable to you. If not, move on to the next stop.
- Eliminate the obvious gluten and ask about ingredients that arouse suspicion. Determine what ingredients might be removed to make a meal safe, such as the croutons on a salad or the bun that goes with a hamburger. If necessary, look at items that could be made gluten-free if only one thing was adjusted, such as substituting a baked potato for French fries or asking to hold the soy sauce-based marinade for meats.
- Let your server know you are gluten-intolerant so they are aware and can provide you the best service they can.
- Inquire about cross-contact to learn if it will be a concern. Provide guidance to the server or management if necessary.
- Consider dining at off-peak times if you can. The slower pace of service can accommodate more interaction with your server and allow for more attention to detail in meeting your requirements.

- Above all, never hesitate to ask for clarification if you are unsure about a dish.

How can you encourage your favorite restaurant to offer gluten-free options?

Restaurants are receiving more gluten-free requests from their customers, but many still don't think the demand warrants creating a gluten-free menu or offering additional gluten-free items. If more gluten-free diners become more vocal about their needs, this may change.

Consider the following tips if you would like a restaurant to offer more gluten-free options:

- Join your local celiac community support group. Share the number of members with restaurant owners, chefs or managers. This number could shed light on a new market they can cater to if they offered gluten-free options. Offer to share information about their new gluten-free menu items with the support group via their newsletter or postings.
- Don't be shy about letting the restaurant know about gluten-free food products that could substitute well for items they have. For example, bring in a package of your favorite gluten-free pasta as an option to consider having on hand to make their traditional spaghetti gluten-free upon request. Or suggest alternative flours such as rice flour or potato starch to use in place of wheat flour for dusting meats.
- Let them know that you would visit their restaurant more often, bring friends and family members with you, and spread the word to the local gluten-free community if they offered more gluten-free items on the menu. After presenting your case, the restaurant may be encouraged to take your advice. More gluten-free diners need to

be vocal about their interests to help restaurateurs take their establishments to the next level of gluten-free diet awareness and service.

Can you eat gluten-free at fast-food restaurants?

Trying to eat gluten-free at most fast-food restaurants is like trying to buy shoes at a drug store—it may be possible, but your options will be extremely limited. Fast-food restaurants mostly serve foods that have wheat as a primary ingredient, and many of the foods are fried, highly processed, and preserved. You can't expect them to offer gluten-free bread for your hamburger, a gluten-free tortilla for your burrito, or gluten-free breading for your fried chicken. A collection of sides or a salad may be all you can expect. You may be able to order certain items without the bun. French fries are likely to be cross-contaminated because of being fried in the same oil as foods with wheat, plus they may contain wheat starch.

Remember that fast-food restaurants will present numerous challenges in finding foods you can eat in addition to presenting a variety of cross-contact issues. But if you choose to make the fast-food gluten-free eating attempt, keep the following pointers in mind:

- The gluten-free ratio will be considerably smaller than the full-service restaurants you have found to be gluten-free friendly.
- Before visiting a fast-food restaurant, visit their Web site to see if they have a gluten-free menu and read the nutritional information they have posted. Of the many large fast-food chains, Wendy's has a rather extensive gluten-free menu.
- If you choose to ask questions, do so inside instead of using the drive thru speaker phone.
- It's unrealistic to ask a fast-food restaurant to conform to your gluten-free diet needs until corporate headquarters or the owner has implemented a process to do so.

Are bakeries off limits?

Most bakeries across the country specialize in baking breads using traditional wheat flour, and the chances of you finding a gluten-free muffin, scone or cookie in a bakery are unfortunately low. Therefore, enter with low expectations and patiently await the day they will be available. In the meantime, an increasing number of foresighted entrepreneurs are opening independent bakeries designed to offer gluten-free baked goods. They recognize the current demand for these items and know it will continue to increase as more Americans adopt a gluten-free diet.

It is becoming more common to find bakeries in large cities that cater exclusively to special diets, generally offering gluten-free, sugar-free, and vegan baked delights. These bakeries may be dedicated gluten-free facilities also, which eliminate concern for cross-contact.

Research which bakeries in your city offer gluten-free items in addition to their traditional baked goods. But with any bakery that is not a dedicated gluten-free facility, be sure to inquire about their procedures on avoiding cross-contact. This is important, particularly if you are sensitive to the slightest trace of gluten. You'll want to know that they use dedicated or thoroughly cleaned equipment for the gluten-free products. Ask them if they bake in dedicated gluten-free ovens, and if not, ask what their cleaning practices are. If you are very sensitive, gluten dust in the air can be enough to trigger a reaction—you should avoid traditional bakeries entirely.

Also, if a bakery buys gluten-free items for their store from another supplier, consider researching the supply source to ensure their ingredients and manufacturing processes meet your standards.

What about coffee shops?

You need to watch out for the beverages in coffee shops. Fresh ground coffee beans that don't have flavor coatings are naturally gluten-free, but you need to watch out for anything added to or already included in a beverage at a coffee shop. In today's coffee-loving world, lengthy beverage menus and near-infinite combinations for designing your personalized perk make avoiding gluten tricky and can be a game of coffee roulette if you're not careful.

You will need to consider every ingredient that is added to your coffee beverage. These ingredients include but are not limited to syrup for flavoring, thickening agents used, ingredients to enhance froth, and whipped cream and non-dairy substitutes. You also need to check the gluten-free status of rice and soy milk—some brands will use barley enzymes in the manufacturing process. Each of these ingredients has the potential for hidden gluten. Instead of researching each ingredient in your drink with a line of customers behind you, ask the barista if they have suggestions for gluten-free beverages. At the very least, they should be able to tell you what ingredients to avoid and then you can design your beverage from there. But if they can't provide the information you need, you're better off ordering a simple beverage you know is gluten-free. Consider calling or e-mailing the corporate headquarters or individual owner to inquire about each ingredient so you'll know what you can have on your next visit.

Typically, regular coffee and espresso without flavorings, lattes and cappuccinos without flavorings, Americano coffee, and regular iced tea without flavorings are all gluten-free.

When should you leave a restaurant?

Sometimes you will be caught in a spontaneous situation where you will not have had an opportunity to research a restaurant before you end up there. These circumstances inevitably result in at least one situation where you will have to leave a restaurant and find another. One or more of these red flags can be good occasion to leave an establishment:

- There is virtually nothing you can eat on the menu except a side of lettuce and water.
- The staff is not knowledgeable about gluten and where it can be found on their menu, or they are not helpful in allowing you to read ingredient lists for certain products in question.
- If you find you are spending more time educating the staff on gluten than you feel you should.
- If the staff is so busy you feel that you are not receiving the proper attention and critical points of service may be missed.
- If you are not confident in the server's ability to communicate your needs to the cook and how to avoid cross-contact.
- When cross-contact issues can't be avoided because of the nature of the equipment they use to prepare the majority of items on the menu, such as deep fryers in fast-food restaurants.
- When you feel that the staff is not taking your situation seriously.
- If the restaurant is also a bakery and your sensitivity to gluten is so high that bakery dust will produce an uncomfortable reaction.

Chapter 11

ETHNIC CUISINES: TIPS FOR RECIPES AND WHAT TO LOOK FOR ON RESTAURANT MENUS

- What are the translations for some gluten-based words in popular foreign languages?
- What are some classic foods that are off-limits in American cuisine? And what can you eat?
- What are some foods that are off-limits in Italian cuisine? And what can you eat?
- What are some foods that are off-limits in Asian cuisine? And what can you eat?
- What are some foods that are off-limits in French cuisine? And what can you eat?
- What are some foods that are off-limits in German cuisine? And what can you eat?
- What are some foods that are off-limits in Mexican cuisine? And what can you eat?
- What are some foods that are off-limits in Indian cuisine? And what can you eat?
- What are some foods that are off-limits in Greek/Meditteranean cuisine? And what can you eat?
- What are some foods that are off-limits in Spanish/Latin cuisine? And what can you eat?
- What are some foods that are off-limits in Scandinavian cuisine? And what can you eat?
- What are some foods that are off-limits in South American cuisine? And what can you eat?
- What are some foods that are off-limits in Eastern European cuisine? And what can you eat?

What are the translations for some gluten-based words in popular foreign languages?

A Crash Course in Gluten Vocabulary:

Italian

Gluten:	Glutine
Bread:	Pane
Flour:	Farine
Wheat:	Frumento
Barley:	Orzo
Rye:	Segale
Oats:	Avena
Pasta:	Pasta

French

Gluten:	Gluten
Bread:	Pain
Flour:	Farine
Wheat:	Blé
Barley:	Orge
Rye:	Seigle
Oats:	Avoine
Pasta:	Pâtes

German

Gluten:	Glueten
Bread:	Brot
Flour:	Mehl
Wheat:	Weizen
Barley:	Gerste
Rye:	Roggen

Oats:	Hafer
Pasta:	Teigwaren

Spanish

Gluten:	Gluten
Bread:	Pan
Flour:	Harina
Wheat:	Trigo
Barley:	Cebada
Rye:	Centeno
Oats:	Avena
Pasta:	Pastas

Swedish

Gluten:	Gluten
Bread:	Bröd
Flour:	Mjöl
Wheat:	Vete
Barley:	Korn
Rye:	Räg
Oats:	Havre
Pasta:	Pasta

What are some classic foods that are off-limits in American cuisine? And what can you eat?

Not only is America a melting pot of culture, it's a melting pot of gluten-laden cuisine with international influences. The United States has its own special blend of gluten-based cuisine that's encyclopedic in scope, but following are some tips for reading menus to eliminate gluten in classic American favorites:

Avoid	Why?
Barbequed meats	Sauce
Beef Wellington	Puff pastry/flour and baked goods
Breads	Flour
Calzones	Flour
Casseroles	Gravy/flour and bread crumbs
Chicken a la king	Flour
Chicken livers	Flour/dusting
Chicken pot pie	crust/flour
Chowder	Flour
Cobbler	Flour
Croutons	Flour
Desserts/pies	Crust and fillings/flour-based cakes
Eggs benedict	Bread/English muffin
Fish fillets/Sticks	Breaded/fried
French fries	Cross-contaminated oil/possible wheat starch
Fried chicken	Batter/flour
Gravy	Flour
Hamburgers	Buns
Meatloaf	Bread crumbs and worcestershire sauce
Macaroni and cheese	Pasta
Oatmeal	Cross-contaminated oats
Pancakes/waffles	Flour
Salad dressings	Wheat flour/starch/soy sauce
Sandwiches	Bread
Sauces	Flour (possible)
Scalloped potatoes	Flour/bread crumbs
Sloppy joes	Buns/barbeque sauce
Stromboli	Flour
Stuffing	Bread

Following are some suggestions where you can find gluten-free meals in American restaurants, but expect to design your own meals often by either selecting sides and putting them together for a meal or making adjustments to make them gluten-free. Of course, always keep cross-contamination issues in mind.

Gluten-free American fare:
Steak and potatoes
Grilled meats and fish without breading, dusting with flour, or dredging in flour
Vegetable and fruit salads
Rice
Salads without croutons
Steamed vegetables

What are some foods that are off-limits in Italian cuisine? And what can you eat?

Gluten is particularly abundant in Italian cuisine. Common ingredients to look out for include but are not limited to:

Pasta
Bread
Bread crumbs
Breaded meats and vegetables
Desserts
Meats dredged in flour
Meats dusted in flour
Sauces

The following list provides an abridged recipe/menu name primer of some popular gluten-based Italian recipes often found on menus in North America and abroad. If you see these names on a menu, you know that dish is to be avoided:

Avoid	Why?
Arangini (Italian rice balls)	Bread crumbs
Bruschetta	Flour/bread toast
Calamari fritti	Fried/breaded
Calzone/stromboli	Flour/bread
Cannoli	Pasta/flour
Chicken Scarpariello	Flour/dredging
Chicken/veal parmesan	Breading
Crostini	Flour/bread
Eggplant parmesan	Breading (possible—inquire)
Fettuccini alfredo	Pasta/flour
Focaccia	Flour/bread
Gnocchi	Flour/pasta
Italian wedding soup	Bread crumbs
Lasagna	Pasta/flour
Manicotti	Flour/pasta
Meatballs	Bread crumbs
Minestrone	Pasta/flour (possible—inquire)
Mornay sauce	Flour/thickener
Pizza	Flour/crust
Ravioli	Flour
Roui	Bread crumbs
Struffoli	Flour
Tarradls	Flour
Tiramisu	Flour
Tortellini	Pasta/flour
Torta	Flour

Even though it may seem as though the above listing of recipes to be avoided eliminates almost everything from Italian cuisine, take solace in knowing that many other Italian dishes can delight you. Keep in mind that many Italian recipes can be made gluten-free simply by substituting gluten-free pasta. Listed are a few examples.

Gluten-free Italian fare:
Carabaccia (without bread)
Castagnaccio (Italian chestnut flour cake)
Eggplant Parmesan (without breading)
Insalata Caprese (mozzarella, tomato, and basil)
Peposo (peppery stew)
Polenta
Risotto
Shrimp scampi
Sufato (stew)
Viligette (beef rolls)
Zuppa Toscana (soup)

What are some foods that are off-limits in Asian cuisine? And what can you eat?

Asia relies more on rice than the cereal grain wheat, but there is still plenty of gluten to avoid. There are a frustrating amount of food items that could be deemed gluten-free if it weren't for soy sauce in the recipe! Soy sauce is found in almost every Asian dish, and it's not the wheat-free version. Taking soy sauce out of Asian cuisine would be like removing tomato sauce from pasta in Italy—nearly impossible. In Asian cuisine, gluten is typically found in but not limited to:

Breaded/floured/wrapped and fried foods
Noodles

Soy sauce and other sauces
Wrappers

The following list provides an abridged recipe/menu name primer of some popular gluten-based Asian dishes often found on menus in North America and abroad. If you see these names on a menu, you know that dish is to be avoided:

Avoid	*Why?*
Dim sum	Flour/wrappers
Cashew chicken	Soy sauce
Chinese dumplings	Flour/wrappers
Chicken teriyaki	Soy sauce
Chow noodles	Fried noodles
Egg rolls	Flour/wrappers
Fried rice	Soy sauce
Fortune cookies	Flour
Noodle soups	Noodles/flour
Panko	Bread crumbs
Pepper steak	Soy sauce
Pot stickers	Flour
Sesame chicken	Soy sauce/flour
Sweet and sour chicken/pork/beef	Soy sauce/wheat and dusting
Tempura	Flour/batter/fried
Wontons	Flour/wrapping
Wonton soup	Flour/wrapping

The good aspect about Asian cuisine is that you can transform so many of its gluten-based dishes into gluten-free versions simply by substituting wheat-free soy sauce for regular sauce, substituting gluten-free rice noodles for wheat-based noodles, and/or substituting potato starch or corn starch for wheat flour in many fried foods that call for dusting meat before frying. Below is just a sampling of some *inherently* gluten-free Asian recipes. When the soy sauce is an accompaniment, substitute for it or leave it out.

Gluten-free Asian fare:
100 percent buckwheat/soba noodles
Cabbage wrapped pork rolls
California rolls
Chinese gau (Dessert)
Egg drop soup
Egg pancakes
Jook (rice pudding)
Kyuri no sunome (Japanese cucumber salad)
Miso soup
Mochi
Pho (Vietnamese beef and noodle soup)
Spring rolls
Sushi

What are some foods that are off-limits in French cuisine? And what can you eat?

The French are also known for an abundance of wheat flour in their cuisine. Common ingredients to look out for include but are not limited to:

Bread
Breaded meats and vegetables
Desserts
Dredging meats in flour
Dusting meats in flour
Sauces

The following list provides an abridged recipe/menu name primer of some popular gluten-based French recipes often found on menus in North America and abroad. If you see these names on a menu, you know that dish is to be avoided:

Avoid	*Why?*
Béchamel sauce	Flour
Beignets	Flour
Beef Bourguignon	Flour
Calfouti	Flour
Cassoulet	Bread crumbs
Chicken/Veal Cordon Bleu	Bread crumbs
Crepes	Flour
Croque-monsieur	Bread and flour
Espagnole sauce	Flour
Far Breton	Flour
Fougasse	Flour
Madeleines	Flour
Pâte à choux	Flour
Roux	Flour
Quiche	Flour
Souffles	Flour
Tarte flambée	Bread dough
Tarts	Flour

French cuisine without flour is like making music without notes—it seems impossible. However, there are a variety of dishes and sauces you can enjoy. Many French recipes can be made gluten-free by eliminating the sauce, although that might seem sacrilegious. For sauces that call for a small amount of flour, try substituting finely sifted white rice flour or a gluten-free starch to create the roux (sauce base).

Gluten-free French fare:
Beuree blanc (butter sauce)
Bouillabaisse
Chicken fricassee
Choucroute
Confit
Crème Anglaise
Crème brûlée
French onion soup (without bread)
Pipérade
Ratatouille
Steak au poivre
Sauce Andalouse

What are some foods that are off-limits in German cuisine? And what can you eat?

Germany is famous for their baked goods and cuisine laden with gluten, making it one of the more challenging cuisines to maneuver around. German baking often uses the term "kuchen" (which means cake), and will differentiate one cake from another with different words attached to kuchen. So, when you see kuchen, and you'll see it often, you'll know it has gluten!

While the tastes of the cuisines are extraordinarily different, the Germans use gluten in a fashion similar to the Italians, except there isn't as much pasta. Some areas you need to avoid:

Bread
Breaded meats and vegetables
Desserts
Meats dredged in flour
Meats dusted with flour

German pasta (spaetzel)
Sauces

The following list provides an abridged recipe/menu name primer of some popular gluten-based German recipes often found on menus in North America and abroad. If you see these names on a menu, you know that dish is to be avoided:

Avoid	Why?
Beef Stroganoff	Bullion/egg noodles
Berlinerkranze	Flour
Dumplings	Flour
German meatballs	Bread crumbs
German potato salad	Flour
Goulash	When served with egg noodles
Griesbrei	Cream of wheat
Jan Hagels	Flour
Kartoffelpuffer	Flour
Kuchen	Flour
Marzipan	Not typically, but can have flour
Maultaschen	Flour/dumplings
Schnitzel	Breading/flour
Spaetzle	Flour
Stollen	Flour
Strudel	Flour
Tartlets	Flour
Tortes	Flour

A variety of German dishes can be transformed into gluten-free versions by substituting gluten-free noodles or pasta for traditional egg noodles. Try replacing the all-purpose flour in German-baked goods recipes with an all-purpose gluten-free flour blend. As the following list reveals, gluten-free German recipes are not as abundant as in other cuisines, but keep looking if you're a fan of the foods from Deutschland.

Goulash (without egg noodles)
Kartoffellpuree (mashed potatoes)
Linsensalat (lentil salad)
Rot Kohl (German red cabbage)
Sauerbraten
Sauerkraut
Zimtstern (with GF almond paste)

What are some foods that are off-limits in Mexican cuisine? And what can you eat?

While Mexican cuisine utilizes wheat flour to a large extent in its Tortillas, Sopaipillas, and Empanadas, the cuisine has a powerful gluten-free contingent when 100 percent corn tortillas are used. While you always have to be cautious of food preparation, in Mexican cuisine it's less common to find the breading, dusting, and dredging with flour that's so common with Italian, French, and German foods. Where tortillas are listed, always use or request 100 percent corn tortillas and you should be okay.

The most common gluten offenders include but are not limited to:

Flour tortillas
Fried foods with tortillas
Desserts

The following list provides an abridged recipe/menu name primer of some popular gluten-based Mexican foods found on menus in

North America and abroad. If you see these names on a menu, you know that dish is to be avoided:

Avoid	*Why?*
Burritos	Flour tortillas
Chiles rellenos	Flour/batter/fried
Chimichangas	Fried flour tortillas
Croquetas	Flour
Empanadas	Flour
Quesadillas	Flour tortillas
Sopaipilla	Flour
Tres leches	Flour

Mexican cuisine offers a variety of recipes that are gluten-free when 100 percent corn tortillas are used. When bread and dessert recipes call for flour, try substituting a cup-for-cup gluten-free replacement flour, or look for versions in gluten-free cookbooks that have been modified appropriately.

Gluten-free Mexican fare:
Albondigas (meatballs)
Carne adovada (pork cubes)
Chile con queso (chile and melted cheese dip)
Chorizo (spicy pork sausage)
Flan (custard)
Frijoles (beans)
Huevos rancheros (use 100 percent corn tortillas)
Menudo (soup)
Nachos (use 100 percent corn tortilla chips)
Refritos (refried beans)
Salsas

Tamales (use 100 percent cornmeal)
Tostadas (use 100 percent corn tortillas)
Enchiladas (use 100 percent corn tortillas)
Tacos (use 100 percent corn taco shells)

What are some foods that are off-limits in Indian cuisine? And what can you eat?

Interestingly, India is not as reliant on wheat and other gluten-based grains as other cultures. Dusting and dredging meats in flour or breading is also not as common. And while Indian cuisine uses wheat flour in a variety of breads and dishes, finding gluten-free foods on menus in Indian restaurants in North America is not as challenging as it can be in other cuisines. Primarily look out for

Breads
Desserts
Breaded meats and vegetables

The following list provides an abridged recipe/menu names primer of some popular gluten-based Indian foods found on menus in North America and abroad. If you see these names on a menu, you know that dish is to be avoided:

Avoid	*Why?*
Aloo ka paratha	Flour
Chapati	Flour
Kesari	Flour
Naan (flat bread)	Flour
Palak vada (dumplings)	Flour
Pooris	Flour
Poulourie	Flour
Roti	Flour

Indian cuisine is known for its heavy use of spices, and much of the cuisine is also vegetarian. One of the most popular dishes is dal, which is made from split gram beans commonly known as lentils. This dish can be made many ways and using many different ingredients and spices. Also, many dishes feature gluten-free flours, particularly besan (or chickpea flour). When eating spices, make sure they are gluten-free.

Gluten-free Indian fare:
Beef vindaloo
Chicken biryani
Chicken pyaza
Chicken masala
Chutneys
Cucumber soup
Coconut barfi (dessert)
Dal (many variations)
Gajar ka halwa (pudding)
Gram flour cakes
Garam masala (sauce)
Khaman dhokla (steamed cake)
Kodbale (crispy rice loops)
Mulligatawny soup
Nippattu (flat bread)
Rasam (soup)
Raita (yogurt)
Saag (spinach dish)
Tandoori chicken

What are some foods that are off-limits in Greek/Mediterranean cuisine?

Unlike Italian and German cuisine, Greek cuisine does not rely as much on pasta/noodles or dredging and dusting meats in flour, yet there is plenty to watch out for. Orzo is the name for Greek pasta, couscous (a wheat pasta) is a regional favorite, and desserts like the famous baklava use phyllo dough, which is far from gluten-free. Common foods to look out for include but are not limited to:

Bread
Orzo
Phyllo dough meat pies
Desserts

The following list provides an abridged recipe/menu names primer of some popular gluten-based Greek or Mediterranean recipes often found on menus in North America and abroad. If you see these names on a menu, you know that dish is to be avoided:

Avoid	*Why?*
Avgolemono	Orzo pasta/flour
Baklava	Flour/phyllo dough
Coquilles	Bread crumbs
Couscous	Wheat
Diples	Flour
Finikia	Flour
Galaktoboureko	Flour
Gyros	Bread/pita
Kotopitta	Flour/phyllo dough
Kreatopitta	Flour/phyllo dough
Moussaka	Flour

Pastitsio	Flour/bread crumbs/pasta
Saganaki	Flour
Spanakopita	Flour/phyllo dough
Tabbouleh	Bulgur wheat (often used)
Taramisalata	Bread used
Tiropitas	Flour

Greek cuisine is famous for using phyllo dough in meat pies, stuffed meats or vegetable pockets, and desserts. And unfortunately anything with phyllo dough must be avoided. But Mediterranean food is revered for its many healthy characteristics, made all the more enjoyable when paired with good wine and conversation! Fortunately, you will find some Greek/Mediterranean specialties to entice and delight your gluten-free palate. Below is a sampling of naturally gluten-free recipes to explore.

Gluten-free Mediterranean fare:
Greek salad
Fasolatha (Greek bean soup)
Souzoukaklia (beef skewers)
Hummus (garbanzo bean dip)
Dolmas (rice-stuffed grape leaves)
Dolmathes (meat and rice-stuffed grape leaves)
Mezethakia (fried cheese squares)
Sheftalia (Greek sausage)
Bourtheto (red fish stew)

What are some foods that are off-limits in Spanish/ Latin cuisine? And what can you eat?

While wheat flour is used in certain Spanish recipes, it's easier to avoid gluten in this cuisine because the culture simply does not use it as prolifically as others do. You will need to primarily watch out for:

Bread
Flour in baked and fried foods
Pasta (fideo—occasionally)

The following list provides an abridged recipe/menu title primer of some popular gluten-based Spanish/Latin recipes containing wheat flour and are more common abroad than in North America. If you see these names on a menu, you know that dish is to be avoided:

Avoid	*Why?*
Churros	Flour
Croquetas	Flour
Empanadas	Flour
Fideo	Flour/pasta
Pan de Horno	Bread
Romesco Sauce	Bread

Spanish/Latin cuisine romances the palate with vibrant flavors. Seafood, rice, vegetables, legumes, and spices are essential to this cuisine, which focuses on fresh ingredients of varying regions. Thankfully, gluten-free options in this cuisine abound.

Gluten-free Spanish/Latin fare:
Almond blancmange (pudding)
Arroz con pollo (chicken and rice)
Black bean soup
Ceviche (seafood salad)

Escabeche (marinated or poached fish)
Gazpacho (cold vegetable soup)
Mole (sauce)
Mojo (sauce)
Natilla (custard)
Paella (rice dish often made with seafood)
Spanish rice
Tapas (minus the pastries)
Tortilla de patatas (potato omelet/tortilla)

What are some foods that are off-limits in Scandinavian cuisine? And what can you eat?

Scandinavian cuisine is rich with seafood as well as such staples as reindeer, venison, and lingonberries. Modern Scandinavian cuisine offers a wealth of delicious recipes without gluten, but their bread, pastries, and desserts are still predominant and unfortunately off-limits for the gluten-free traveler. In Scandinavian cuisine, gluten is largely found in but not limited to:

Bread
Desserts
Many meat-based entrees

The list below mentions just a few gluten-based foods among hundreds you can expect to find in Scandinavia, some of which are enjoyed in North America (such as Swedish meatballs). Unfortunately, these Nordic delicacies are unsafe unless, of course, they are transformed into gluten-free versions:

Avoid	*Why?*
Canapes	Toppings placed on bread
Open faced sandwiches	Toppings placed on bread

Kringle	Flour
Norwegian lefse	Bread crumbs/flour
Norwegian skolebrod	Flour
Swedish limpa	Bread
Swedish meatballs	Bread crumbs
Swedish pancakes	Flour
Swedish klimp	Flour
Wienerbrød (Danishes)	Bread

When you navigate around the multitude of pastries found in this beautiful region, you'll find a variety of dishes that capture the essence of the cuisine without the gluten. Listed are a few naturally gluten-free, old-world recipes from Scandinavia to explore on your gluten-free journey.

Gluten-free Scandinavian fare:
Canapes (toppings are gluten-free without the bread)
Gravlax (raw cured salmon without the bread)
Pickled herring
Swedish julgrot (rice pudding)
Portketta (pork roast)
Riisivanukas (Finnish rice pudding)
Pasha (Finnish Easter dessert)
Kaalikääryleet (meat and rice stuffed cabbage rolls—hold the gravy)
Brunede Kartofler (Danish sugar browned potatoes)

What are some foods that are off-limits in South American cuisine? And what can you eat?

South American cuisine is a melting pot of different cultural influences from Argentina, Brazil, and Venezuela to Peru, Uruguay, Chile, and several other countries. For the gluten-free traveler, options in this cuisine genre are delightfully abundant. Wheat flour, while used, comprises a relatively small portion of their recipes in general. Primarily, be on the look out for bread crumbs and flour in bread-like goods.

The following list provides an abridged recipe/menu name primer of some popular gluten-based South American recipes. By no means a comprehensive list, the small number listed reveals that flour is not a main staple in this cuisine. If you see these names on a menu, you know that dish is to be avoided:

Avoid	*Why?*
Albondiguitas	Bread crumbs
Bolo Bebado	Flour
Bunuelos	Flour
Churros	Flour
Empanadas	Flour
Matambre	Bread crumbs

In comparison to the foods you must avoid, your chances of finding naturally gluten-free recipes from South America far outnumber those with gluten. Have fun exploring this cuisine because it has so many options for the gluten-free gourmet. Listed here are just a few recipes to pique your interest.

Gluten-free South American fare:
Anticuchos (Peruvian beef kebabs)
Brigadeiro (Brazilian fudge)
Chimichurri (Argentinean sauce)
Feijoada (Brazilian black bean stew)
Moqueca de peixe (fish stew)

Pabellon criollo (Venezuelan steak)
Pao de queijo (Brazilian cheese bread rolls)
Pastel de choclo (Chilean corn pie)
Pebre (Chilean hot pepper sauce)
Salpicao (Brazilian chicken salad)
Sancocho (chicken stew)
Sopa Paraguaya (Paraguayan cheese cornbread)
Tostones (fried plantains)

What are some foods that are off-limits in Eastern European cuisine? And what can you eat?

When traveling to Europe, your experience in dodging gluten will be rather similar to what you find in North America—it's everywhere! While in cuisines like South American and Indian you can find a variety of dishes that incorporate meat, fish, and vegetables without sneaking in flour, it's more challenging to find European dishes without at least a tablespoon or more of flour. Generally, however, substituting a nice finely ground rice flour will suffice without dramatically altering the chemistry and taste of the recipe. Everywhere you will have to watch for the following:

Bread
Bread crumbs
Flour
Pasta/noodles
Desserts

The following list provides an abridged recipe/menu name primer of some popular gluten-based Eastern European recipes. If you see these names on a menu, you know that dish is to be avoided:

Avoid	*Why?*
Blini	Flour
Goulash	Flour
Kugel	Noodles/flour
Kulich	Flour
Kutia	Barley
Latkes	Flour
Lebkuchen	Flour
Linzertorte	Flour
Moussaka	Bread crumbs
Pierogies	Flour
Rugelach	Flour
Spaetzle	Flour/pasta
Stroganoff	Flour/noodles
Topfenknodel	Flour
Truklji	Flour

Unfortunately, finding a wide variety of naturally gluten-free recipes in Eastern Europe is a challenge. While there are many more than those contained in the following list, you can tell that this is not the most gluten-free friendly cuisine. If this genre of food is enticing to you, consider making many meat and gravy-based recipes gluten-free by using a rice flour or gluten-free starch in a sauce or gravy recipe that calls for wheat. And when noodles are called for, consider substituting gluten-free pasta or noodles, or even rice.

Gluten-free Eastern European fare:
Borscht (soup)
Charoset (dessert)
Kasha (roasted buckwheat)

Paprikash (meat dish—hold the noodles)
Shepherd's pie
Uborkasalata (cucumber salad)

Chapter 12

TRAVELING: MAKING TRIPS WORRY- AND HUNGER-FREE

■ What is some good advice for dining out when on a long road trip?

■ What should you always take with you when traveling?

■ Can you eat gluten-free at airports?

■ Will airplanes have gluten-free meals?

■ What should you know about staying in a hotel?

■ What should you know about staying at a bed-and-breakfast or lodge?

■ Should you avoid vending machines?

■ How can you best prepare for international travel?

■ Which countries are more aware of gluten-intolerance?

■ What should you do when dining out in a foreign country?

■ What happens if you can't get past a language barrier?

■ How can you avoid cross-contamination when traveling abroad?

■ How do you eat gluten-free at business events when traveling?

■ How can you improve your gluten-free diet when traveling?

■ Who can help you with your gluten-free travel arrangements and logistics?

■ What snacks are good while traveling by plane?

What is some good advice for dining out on a long road trip?

Many of the rules you follow for dining out on a long road trip are similar to the ones you use at home (Chapter Nine)—however, expect the challenge to be turned up several notches. We're all too familiar with the sudden exhaustion and hunger that can overwhelm us on the road, teasing our temper and increasing the desperation to eat to a level where we're tempted to consume something irresponsible. You want to avoid hitting this point, then having to wander around in an unfamiliar city trying to find something you can eat. Aimlessness can cloud your judgment and weaken your willpower— plan ahead to avoid doing something unsafe.

Begin by mapping out your route at home, then research the restaurant scene in the cities you'll be traveling through and go ahead of time to find the options you can live with. Submit a post to the online celiac community asking if anyone knows of a gluten-free friendly restaurant in the city you need. Your strategy for both small and large cities will be the same, but expect the ratio of options to decrease in small towns. If the dining options in a city don't yield to what you're looking for, always be able and willing to shop for foods you can eat at a grocery store and eat in your car or hotel room, or subsist on the foods you brought with you.

Tip: Look for natural foods stores when researching your cities. These stores cater to the natural food customer, many of whom purchase gluten-free products, and it's possible there will be dining options nearby that follow suit because of the local market demand. Conversely, if the town does not have a natural foods store, it might be harder to find gluten-free dining options as well. And most importantly, never leave home without a plan and some gluten-free food!

What should you always take with you when traveling?

Traveling gluten-free requires a set of rules and guidelines—take just one trip with several pitfalls and disappointments, and you'll draft a checklist of things to remember for your next trip. The following tips, strategies, and suggestions will help you avoid many of the common mistakes and disappointments of inexperienced gluten-free travelers. But first, remember that aside from the standard guidelines and rules that come with every gluten-free trip, you need to always arm yourself with five things before ever leaving the house, whether it is for business or pleasure: a plan, realistic expectations, flexibility, thinking outside the box, and willpower.

- Keep in mind that dining out may not always be the best option, so shopping at grocery stores and eating in your car or taking food back to your hotel room may be a safer and healthier option.
- *Always* bring some gluten-free food with you. Car trips have more available space, while airplane trips are more limiting, but carrying your snacks in baggies to eliminate boxes will save space. These snacks will often be lifesavers, and they may occasionally serve as meal replacements when gluten-free options are not as available as you would like.
- When new to the gluten-free lifestyle, reference tools can help you avoid mistakes, save time and eliminate frustration, particularly when hunger and desperation kick in. Bring ingredient lists on cards that can fit inside your wallet for quick reference.
- Have with you the contact information from the local celiac/gluten-intolerance support group in the cities where you are traveling.
- If you're staying in a condo with a kitchen, bring a good supply of groceries from home and eat there. Plan your meals ahead.

This saves time, money, research, and a lot of guesswork.

- Have notes and phone numbers for restaurants you have queried ahead of time for gluten-free menu options.

Can you eat gluten-free at airports?

It's possible to eat gluten-free at airports, but gluten reigns supreme for the typical hungry traveler and it's wise to expect less than abundant options. Whether large or small, airports are designed to cater to the fast-paced traveler quickly and efficiently with menu items that typically don't meet special dietary needs.

With busy travelers standing in line behind you, asking if something is gluten-free and avoiding cross-contact will often throw a curve ball at the staff behind the register. The pressure from the people waiting behind you, generally in a hurry to get somewhere, can force you into making decisions that may not be in your self-interest, particularly if you're hungry and running short on time too.

Pressed for time? When dining at an airport restaurant, keep in mind that your special dietary requests or meal modifications can take a long time to accommodate and leave you with not enough time to eat comfortably and make it to your flight. Dine with realistic expectations and expect most of your menu options to revolve around salads.

Bottom Line: Don't rely on airport food to give you the meal you crave for. Be proactive in eating well before you arrive at the airport. Eat a good meal consisting of a nutritious combination of high-quality protein and carbohydrates to keep you feeling satisfied as long as possible. And bring nutritious gluten-free snacks with you!

Tip: If you must eat at an airport, plan to eat light. Unfortunately, because of limited options, salads are your best options at airports. Ask them to hold the croutons and bring your own salad dressing if you can. Salad dressing in mini sealed packets are standard at airports, and the list of ingredients may easily contain gluten.

Will airplanes have gluten-free meals?

Airplanes do not typically serve gluten-free meals. All meals for a flight are produced in mass well in advance, and requesting a gluten-free meal during the flight will not yield much favorable results. A gluten-free meal must be arranged well in advance— many airlines will do their best to accommodate your dietary requests if you follow their policy, but expect to give at least three days advance notice.

Airlines are familiar with providing Kosher and vegetarian options and the gluten-free request is becoming more popular; as long as your request is in place with plenty of time, your chances of getting a safe meal are pretty high. However, always have a backup plan in case your request didn't get communicated properly and you're left flying without anything to eat. As always, make sure you have some gluten-free snacks with you.

Map out the legs of your trip with all stops, request your meals accordingly, and bring enough snacks to either augment your meal or serve as a replacement in case of a mistake with the airline arrangements. Remember that it is common to underestimate your hunger when traveling and you may not bring enough food with you to get you through the trip. Bringing more than you think you'll need is wise.

What should you know about staying in a hotel?

Until coffee shops in hotels start offering gluten-free baked goods, you need to concern yourself primarily with what goes on in the hotel restaurant and the lounge. As with any restaurant, you will need to apply your menu reading skills, watch out for cross-contact issues and have your questions ready. But in hotels, it's wise to be aware of the overall service environment that can make eating gluten-free challenging, particularly if you're under a time constraint.

Hotels are typically bustling places that cater to the on the go business travelers and tourists. Service is particularly fast-paced in the morning. There is one key difference between hotel dining and dining in a free-standing restaurant: hotel chefs and service staff are often serving dining guests simultaneously with room service demands and possibly other restaurants in the hotel, plus the lounge. Special dietary requests can challenge the busy service staff, and service may not be as timely and precise as it could be. So, while asking questions is always a good thing to do, when staying in hotels you may find it better to keep your questions to a minimum and order what you know to be safe. Too many questions could make for an uncomfortable delay, particularly if you have a flight to catch.

Be aware that the level of gluten-free awareness in hotels will vary dramatically. Hotels at Walt Disney World Resorts and Yosemite National Park, for example, are leaders in the special diet arena. Other hotels are easing into it more slowly. Don't expect a hotel to have gluten-free bread for your morning toast, and if they do, remember to ask if they have dedicated toasters for the bread! The Broadmoor in Colorado Springs, Colorado has gluten-free bread at the ready for diners.

What should you know about staying at a bed-and-breakfast or lodge?

At small, intimate lodging such as a bed-and-breakfast, meals are often designed ahead of time and a menu may be in place for the duration of your visit before you even arrive. But fortunately, because of the high level of personalized service often found at a bed-and-breakfast, talking with your hosts can ensure a good, safe experience. B&Bs are known for serving a continental-style breakfast— muffins, fruit, and coffee for all guests. However, these days it's rare that an innkeeper has not received a gluten-free diet request and they have probably made some accommodations, whether it is offering ready-to-eat gluten-free products or recipes created from scratch in preparation for a gluten-free guest.

Research B&Bs that are gluten-free friendly, and let your innkeeper know about your gluten-free and other dietary needs when you make a reservation so they can plan for your arrival. Levels of awareness in B&Bs are improving, but expect it to vary between B&B and from city to city. Communication is the key, and you should be ready to explain your diet and let your host know what you can and can't eat. Also, don't forget to mention cross-contact concerns.

Should you avoid vending machines?

Unless you're familiar with the ingredients and gluten-free status of a product before popping in your change, it's best to save your money; chances are likely that the majority of snacks in a vending machine will contain gluten or were manufactured with products that contain gluten. Naturally, it's impossible to read the ingredient labels behind the glass prior to purchasing, and of all the dangerous aspects of traveling, the vending machine is one area where you can easily avoid the risk.

With a bit of creativity, you can bring your own vending machine snacks with you on the trip. Before leaving home, think about how you can make foods that mimic the appeal of the machine snacks. Consider making your own gluten-free trail mix that has that sweet and salty sensation that vending machine products are famous for. Combining a gluten-free chocolate bar, raisins, or package of nuts can often keep larger cravings at bay. Unless you are sure about certain products, it's best to avoid both the vending and beverage machine.

How can you best prepare for international travel?

The only means to satisfaction and safety during international travel is through plenty of training and practice on the home front, with weeks of research and planning before leaving home. Realize that being weary and unfamiliar with the culture and language at the same time may add additional stress to an already challenging situation. Expect to take everything you have learned at home up by several notches and allow yourself as much research and planning time for your trip as you can before leaving for the airport.

Some key things to remember or consider include:

- Before you board the international flight you'll be asked to discard any unpackaged foods you have because of International Customs food laws. Confirm what you can bring with the airline in advance.
- Consult with gluten-free people who have earlier traveled to your destination and gather tips borne of experience.
- If you're traveling to a non-English speaking country, bring easily accessible premade reference tools that will make reading menus, communicating with service staff, and deciphering food product labels easier and more efficient. Create a list of ingredients and hidden gluten culprits you must avoid and translate them into the foreign language you need. For example, the German words for wheat, barley, and rye are Weizen, Gerste, and Roggen. Also, create a list of key questions in the foreign language. Consult with a professor or student for accuracy, or read *Let's Eat Out* by the founders of GlutenFree Passport for guidelines and information. They've done much of the work for you. And don't forget the dictionary!
- Consider shipping a box filled with your favorite gluten-free products to your destination days in advance.

Which countries are more aware of gluten-intolerance?

While awareness of celiac disease and gluten-intolerance continues to build internationally, some countries that are generally more aware of the condition include Canada, England, Ireland, Italy, New Zealand, and Australia. Italy screens children for celiac disease at an early age and it's not uncommon to find gluten-free pasta in restaurants upon request. In addition to having national support organizations similar to those found in the United States, these countries also have a variety of food manufacturers that specialize in dedicated gluten-free foods, many of which can be found in stores throughout America as well as being available online.

What should you do when dining in a foreign country?

When dining in a non-English speaking country, it's wise to be as familiar as possible with the key gluten-related words, ingredients, phrases and questions in the foreign language. If you're not familiar with the language, some study before you leave home will build your awareness and confidence.

Watch out for processed foods and those made from a recipe. Where there is more than one ingredient in a menu item, there could be gluten. Watch for things such as preserved meats, sauces, gravies, breading, and meat or fish dusted with flour. Prepare yourself to ask basic questions of your server in their language to clarify ingredients and cross-contact issues. Learn how to explain what gluten is in their language, and what it is that you must avoid.

Allow for more time to read and understand the menu. If possible, research restaurants in the vicinity of your lodging accommodations and look at their online menus if available. This will give you practice in scanning menus in a foreign language and can let you know which dishes to avoid before arriving.

Familiarize yourself with the cuisine of the country before traveling. Learn about traditional dishes that are naturally gluten-free (Chapter Ten).

What happens if you can't get past a language barrier?

It's just realistic to expect that this can happen and will be a tough situation. Therefore, always have a backup plan or two in mind. For example, as gluten-free dining options may be scarce, always be on the look out for a grocery store or market near your hotel, or ask for the nearest one when you check in. This can be a lifesaver in tough situations. You'll typically be able to find something you can eat at a store, particularly natural, unprocessed foods like fruits, vegetables, and nuts which can be stored in your hotel using a portable cooler if necessary. Stop by a market and purchase foods that you can have at your hotel in case any of your dining adventures leave you hungry.

If reading a menu is too complicated and frustrating, ask if they can make you something special that includes ingredients and foods from the menu you can eat. While experiencing a variety of dining options is part of the fun in traveling, be prepared and willing to revisit restaurants more than once if you know they can cater to your needs.

Bottom line: Psychologically prepare yourself for possible encounters with language barriers. By being open to this expectation, you can become proactive and look for alternative plans that can get you out of difficult situations.

How can you avoid cross-contamination when traveling abroad?

International travel naturally presents an inherent challenge to gluten-free living because of unfamiliarity, different cultural customs, and the everpresent language barrier. To avoid cross-contamination when abroad, you have to carefully guard your safety, know the questions to ask, and be prepared to educate service staff when necessary. If you employ the skills that you have learned and practiced on the home front for avoiding cross-contamination, your chances for a safe experience abroad increase substantially.

First, never assume anything and always double-check everything. Although it can be challenging, try to know the names of the ingredients you can't have in the foreign language for efficiently scanning menus. Then you'll need to be prepared how to ask about cross-contact well enough in the country's native language to steer you clear. Ask how the foods you are considering will be prepared and be on the look out for techniques such as dusting and dredging meats with flour. This is why having a general knowledge of how many foods are prepared can be beneficial, particularly overseas.

Another good tactic for avoiding cross-contamination is to ask that foods be prepared minimally and separate from other ingredients that can be questionable. And confirm that the service staff understands exactly what you need by having them repeat back to you in their words how they will prepare your meal. Even though you may find certain cities to be quite accommodating to your needs and know how to avoid cross-contact, you need to be prepared for the times when awareness of the issue is not what it should be. Backcountry inns where the staff doesn't speak your language are more prone to communication barriers. But regardless of where you are when abroad, your strategy and safety net boils down to how many questions you're willing and able to ask to protect yourself and with the preparation you have done at home to learn the language and prepare or buy reference lists.

How do you eat gluten-free at business events when traveling?

With the large sit-down banquets or buffets generally found at national business events such as conventions, conferences, and awards-dinners, the meals are typically mass prepared and plated in advance. You will only know what the fare is once it's served or unveiled at the buffet station. It's optimal to connect with the meeting planner of the event weeks ahead of time and ask if there is a way to accommodate your gluten-free needs. If they know in advance and can do something about it, they will be more than happy to do so. However, you should still double-check the day of the event to ensure your request has been processed and was not lost in the shuffle.

But what is your plan B? You need one. Consider eating before you attend a meal event and know that the salad course (hold the croutons!) may have to suffice, or expect to wait to eat until the event is over.

If the business event is being organized by your company, encourage that a caterer with experience in accommodating special diets is selected to bid on the job. There are generally several types of dietary restrictions in an office, and other associates and attendees will be thankful for this accommodation too.

How can you improve your gluten-free diet when traveling?

Whether for business or pleasure, traveling comes with an inherent element of stress and healthy eating will benefit you in more ways than one. But when we're in unfamiliar territory, hustling to make planes, reading maps, and keeping an eye on our belongings, it's easy to overlook our nutritional needs and just look to serve the hunger, not the body. Gluten-free eating does not necessarily mean healthy eating and by the time we're aware of not feeling our best, it's often too late. But there are three tips that can help:

From the start, make sure you're paying attention to fiber. If watching your fiber intake at home is challenging, keeping track on the road is even more so, and traveling can easily disrupt regularity. The gluten-free snacks you bring with you may be sweet, indulgent carbohydrates that keep you happy and full, but may be highly refined and lack quality fiber. So it's important to eat plenty of fresh fruits, vegetables, and salads as much as you can in conjunction with meals and snacks. Adding healthy whole grains such as brown rice can be beneficial also. For every one or two gluten-free carbohydrate snacks you eat, have a fresh fruit like an apple to keep things in balance.

When traveling in planes and cars for long periods of time, water retention is a common complaint. Avoid large amounts of salty and processed gluten-free foods to help keep water retention and bloating from escalating. Consider bringing a small, plastic travel bottle filled with olive oil to use as a healthy salad dressing with lemon—great for eating salads at airports.

And it goes without saying . . . drink plenty of water!

Who can help you with your gluten-free travel arrangements and logistics?

While nothing can replace taking some time to prepare and research your eating options and strategies, thankfully there are companies who have done much of the legwork for the gluten-free traveler and offer educational products, tools, and services that can make traveling and dining more efficient, safe, and enjoyable.

Another passport you'll need . . .

GlutenFree Passport provides educational books and pocket guides for the gluten-free diner and traveler with its award-winning series:

Let's Eat Out! The book covers different cuisines and can be useful wherever you travel. Plus, they offer Multi-Lingual Phrase Passports with French, German, Italian, and Spanish translations that provide easy reference for the questions you need, plus helpful word translations and phrases. To learn more visit www.glutenfreepassport.com.

Where can you eat?

Triumph Dining offers *The Essential Gluten-Free Restaurant Guide*, which outlines hundreds of restaurants throughout the United States that either offer gluten-free menus, have an abundance of gluten-free options on the menu, or have staff that are willing and able to accommodate the gluten-free diner. The company also offers Dining Cards in different cuisines that not only help define what you need to avoid at restaurants but can be useful for giving chefs more information to help serve you best. To learn more visit www.triumphdining.com.

Gluten-Free Getaways

Founded by a husband and wife team, Bob and Ruth's Gluten-Free Dining & Travel Club provides workshops on gluten-free dining and travel in connection with celiac community support groups across the country. They also organize full-scale international trips and mini-getaways throughout the United States and handle all logistics for the group; you simply can relax and enjoy. To learn more visit www.bobandruths.com.

What snacks are good while traveling by plane?

For good gluten-free snacking throughout your trip, rule number one is to bring a little more than you think you'll need or want. It's always better to have too many snacks than too few. Underestimating how hungry you will be in between meals is common among busy travelers, and you need to have enough on you to beat both snacking urges and to serve as a meal if you face trouble finding a safe place to eat. Because airport travel is typically the most challenging, consider the following non-refrigerated snacks, most of which can be carried in resealable baggies:

- Carbo-fuel: Gluten-free crackers, cookies, crisp breads, low-salt chips, cold cereals, rice cakes, and fresh baked goods from home like mini-muffins or brownies
- Fresh fiber: Carrots, celery, zucchini, and strawberries
- Sweet fiber bites: Dried fruits such as apricots, figs, dates, raisins, and prunes
- Fresh fruits: Apples, oranges, pears, grapes, bananas, peaches, and nectarines
- Protein power: Nuts such as almonds, peanuts, and cashews; pumpkin seeds; gluten-free beef or bison jerky
- Mini-meals: Sandwiches made with nut butters and preserves
- Bars away: Individually wrapped, gluten-free nutrition/breakfast bars and chocolates that can easily be stuffed into pockets and purses

Tip: Always bring a healthy combination of carbohydrates, protein, and fiber—all three work together better to fight hunger than just one alone. Your body will appreciate it.

For the suitcase: Pack more of the same goodies as above into your suitcase, as well as packaged or canned fruits, instant gluten-free cereal packets to combine with hot water, and gluten-free rice noodle bowls. Don't forget plastic silverware!

Chapter 13

BAKING AND COOKING: MAKING TRANSITIONS

- How do you begin baking gluten-free?
- What ingredients are commonly used in gluten-free baking?
- What are the different gluten-free flours and starches?
- Can you use just rice flour as a replacement for wheat flour?
- What is a gluten-free flour blend?
- What are some good flour blend formulas for wheat flour substitution?
- Why are certain gluten-free baked goods often dry and crumbly?
- Why do gluten-free baked goods often taste different from wheat-baked goods?
- What improves the texture of gluten-free baked goods?
- What improves moisture content of gluten-free baked goods?
- Are gums required for gluten-free baking?
- What are some easy recipe substitutions to make a traditional recipe gluten-free?
- What are some gluten-free cookbooks?
- What are some websites where I can find gluten-free recipes?
- Are some pieces of equipment better than others for gluten-free baking?
- Can a bread machine make gluten-free bread?

How do you begin baking gluten-free?

Before taking the plunge into the basics of gluten-free baking, you'll need four things: an open mind for learning new methods, a flexible palate for trying new tastes and textures, an adventurous spirit, and a bit of patience. These traits will serve you well from the start, because gluten-free baking is a 180 degree turn from traditional baking. Starting out with a mindset that accepts a different approach will help you enjoy this new journey of tastes and methods as well as help prevent occasional bouts of discouragement or outright disappointment along the way.

Whether you prefer baking from scratch, a packaged mix, or a combination of both, gluten-free baking requires three major paradigm shifts in your thinking about baking:

Paradigm Shift #1: Using single all-purpose flour for each of your baking needs is replaced by using a "flour blend" that combines two or more different gluten-free flours that work in harmony with each other to replicate the wheat-flour effect in baking.

Paradigm Shift #2: Say good-bye to kneading. Gluten-free breads are made from batters similar to cake batters. They are mixed with spoons or paddles and are baked in loaf pans with walls.

Paradigm Shift #3: Gluten gives flexibility to dough and helps bind it together. Gluten-free baking requires key ingredients that replace the gluten to help give structure to the dough; otherwise, the baked goods will fall apart.

What ingredients are commonly used in gluten-free baking?

While traditional baking revolves around wheat flour, successful gluten-free baking utilizes a variety of different flours blended in various combinations. Rice flour is a foundational ingredient in the majority of gluten-free baked goods. The flours made from rice include white rice flour, sweet white rice flour, and brown rice flour. However, rice flour is rarely used alone as a substitute for wheat flour. It's common to find that flour blends combine one or more varieties of rice flour with other "white" flours, typically potato flour and tapioca starch. These ingredients create a blend that helps replace all-purpose wheat flour.

You'll find these flours used in different ratios in both recipes and packaged products. It's nice to have these individual flours on hand in your kitchen. However, you will also find other flours widely used in combination with rice flour, including sorghum flour, soy flour, bean flours and lesser known flours with wonderful baking powers made from nutritious grains including amaranth, buckwheat, quinoa and teff.

In addition to the flours and starches of gluten-free baking, xanthan gum and guar gum are regularly used to help replace the extendibility of gluten and provide the binding structure in a gluten-free baked good. When dampened, these gums provide viscosity and binding properties for blending the flours together and making a gluten-free dough or batter.

What are the different gluten-free flours and starches?

Gluten-free flours come from a variety of sources including rice, other grains, nuts, seeds, and beans. They vary in color, taste, texture, and levels of protein, fiber and other nutrients, as well as culinary and baking performance characteristics. Many of these flours come in organic versions also. Some flours are also referred to as a "meal," which have a courser ground texture with higher moisture content than flour.

Gluten-free flours are usually found in natural food stores both large and small, online malls, individual product manufacturers, and

Asian food markets. Also, starches provide essential properties and work well in combination with flours, but are not used by themselves as a substitute for flour in baking

Flours

Almond Meal/Flour:

Made from raw almonds that have been blanched, this nutty flour is packed with protein and flavor. Particularly well suited for making sweet delights such as cakes, cookies, sweet breads, and an array of desserts.

Amaranth Flour:

Ground from the hearty, nutritious South American grain amaranth, this flour boasts of a nice protein content and is recommended to be used with other gluten-free flours and starches for baking breads.

Black Bean Flour:

This robust flour lends itself well for culinary uses that have Mexican and South American influence as well as vegetarian concoctions.

Brown Rice Flour:

Look for brown rice flour with a fine grind to avoid grittiness. Best used in conjunction with other gluten-free flours for baking.

Buckwheat Flour:

Known for its unique flavor that gives buckwheat pancakes a signature flavor, this flour is particularly high in protein and works well as a complementary flour for baking.

Chestnut Flour:
For sumptuous gluten-free pastries, Italian chestnut flour is a delightful flour with a particularly sweet and nutty flavor. The Italian cake, Castagnaccio, uses this flour exclusively.

Coconut Flour:
This sweet, nutritious flour is high in fiber and is a good source of protein. Enhances baked goods with a rich texture and imparts a distinguishable coco-nutty flavor.

Fava Bean Flour:
Fava beans, a part of the pea family, are found in Mediterranean and Chinese cuisine. Finely ground flour from the fava can be a unique addition for gluten-free cooking and baking.

Flaxseed Meal:
Known for being high in omega 3 fatty acids and fiber, flaxseed meal is a favorable option for adding nutrition to gluten-free baked goods. Use in small amounts. A little goes a long way.

Garbanzo Bean Flour:
The garbanzo bean is widely featured throughout Middle Eastern cuisine and is often found in gluten-free flour blends as a complementary flour.

Green Pea Flour:
A nice option for culinary uses such as thickening a creamy pea soup. This can also be a nice addition to incorporate into gluten-free baked goods as a complementary flour.

Hazelnut Meal/Flour:
This nutritious flour made from freshly ground hazelnuts has a sweet, nutty flavor and is well suited for using in sweet baked goods, similar to how almond flour would be used.

Indian Ricegrass/ Montina:
Particularly high in fiber, this is a robust flour that is used in combination with other flours or as a flavorful, nutritious supplement for gluten-free baking. Once an important staple to the Native American diet, Indian ricegrass has made a comeback via the growing gluten-free food industry.

Mesquite Flour:
Made from succulent bean pods of the mesquite tree, this particularly sweet, richly-colored flour is known for its nutrient-density and low-glycemic index. Brings a distinctive flavor to baked goods when used in small quantities.

Millet Flour:
Yellow in color and subtle in flavor, millet flour is a versatile flour for gluten-free baking and is used in conjunction with other gluten-free flours to not only boost nutrition and flavor but also adds beautiful color.

Millet Meal:
Heartier in texture than millet flour, the meal can enhance texture and flavor for gluten-free whole grain breads.

Potato Flour:
Unlike potato starch, potato flour is a highly transitional flour suitable for baking and cooking. A foundational ingredient in

gluten-free flour blends and great for thickening gravies, soups, and sauces.

Quinoa Flour:
This nutritious flour, similar to amaranth flour, plays a leading role among gluten-free baked goods because of its favorable protein properties and for mimicking the "gluten" factor. Can be used as a full-replacement for wheat flour depending on the recipe but is typically best when used in combination with other gluten-free flours for baking.

White Rice Flour:
Widely used in conjunction with potato flour and tapioca flour, this flour was a pioneering ingredient in gluten-free baking and is still widely used in a multitude of gluten-free goods including Asian noodles.

Sweet White Rice Flour:
Sticky by nature, this flour is glutinous in texture and is prized for enhancing the binding qualities of gluten-free baked goods when used in conjunction with other gluten-free flours.

Sweet White Sorghum Flour:
Known for having properties closest to wheat flour, sorghum flour is particularly favored for its high protein content that helps give baked goods their structure and imparts great flavor. Used in combination with other gluten-free flours, sorghum, also known as milo, is becoming a leading ingredient in gluten-free baking.

Soy Flour:

High in protein, soy flour is often found in gluten-free flour blends for baking despite the strong flavor it imparts. Not recommended to be used by itself as a replacement for wheat flour.

Tapioca Flour:

Made from the South American tuber root manioc (or also known as cassava or yucca), tapioca flour is a staple ingredient in gluten-free baking. Neutral in flavor and not particularly nutritious by itself, this flour shines as an ingredient to help add chewiness to baked goods. Used in the delicious South American cheese bread rolls, Pao de Quejo.

Teff Flour:

Made from the smallest grain in the world native to northern Africa, teff is a high-protein flour with a unique flavor. Can be used in combination with other gluten-free flours in baking to help give structure to baked goods such as cookies and breads.

White Bean Flour:

This nutritious, low-glycemic flour is a versatile culinary ingredient for thickening soups and sauces. Also shines in its ability to bring a lift to gluten-free baked goods when used in conjunction with other flours.

Starches

Arrowroot Starch:

Used primarily as a thickener, the flavor of arrowroot starch is completely neutral and it will not impart an "off" flavor to your recipes. Becomes translucent when cooked and for this reason it can be great for dessert sauces because of its beautiful glossy appearance. But beware. The starch can make your meat sauce have a gluey, fake appearance.

Cornstarch:
Valued for its thickening properties, cornstarch is widely found in creamy products like puddings and soups. To avoid clumping, the starch is often combined with liquid such as water, shaken to create a slurry, and then added to the food to thicken.

Potato Starch:
Not used alone, this starch is favored for its ability to bring moistness to gluten-free baked goods. Also, it is a suitable replacement for wheat flour in thickening gravies, sauces, soups, and stews.

Can you use just rice flour as a replacement for wheat flour?

When first learning how to bake with gluten-free flours, rice flour is a trusty, reliable ingredient, but using just rice flour is rather elementary when turning traditional baking recipes into gluten-free versions. If anything, it's a short-term quick fix to satisfy the cravings when desperation kicks in. But chances are you won't use rice flour by itself for long. However, keep in mind that there are benefits of using only rice flour.

You will soon discover the properties of rice flour and how your baked goods will react and you will likely not be all that pleased. Rice flour does not have the protein content and extendibility characteristics of wheat flour with gluten, and you'll quickly find that your chocolate-chip cookies look flat and crumble in your hands after baking. However, don't consider starting out by baking only with rice flour a waste of time. You'll learn what makes traditional baking different from gluten-free baking, and you'll discover what rice flour can and can't do. As you become more accustomed to the needs of your diet, you'll be able to experiment with different gluten-free flours and blends to find a taste, performance quality, and consistency you like.

What is a gluten-free flour blend?

Saying good-bye to all-purpose wheat flour means entering the world of gluten-free flour blends. Flour is of course elemental to baking, but unlike traditional baking, gluten-free baking does not utilize just one flour. Rather, different flours are used together to achieve better results than what one gluten-free flour can do alone.

A gluten-free flour blend is a combination of two or more gluten-free flours in varying ratios depending upon the purpose you want to achieve. While a gluten-free flour blend can be created that replaces all-purpose wheat flour cup-for-cup, it's more common to experiment with different flours and ratios until you find a unique blend that works in a particular recipe.

Not all gluten-free flour blends are created equal—every gluten-free flour or starch has its own set of characteristics and culinary powers. Some flours are higher in protein and fiber, while some have strong flavors or courser textures. One gluten-free flour blend may work great for a bread and muffin but not so well for another baking and cooking purpose. In fact, different flour blends are often created specifically for the product or recipe in mind. Some flours are used to build structure, and add protein and nutrients, while other flours are used to add a characteristic like improved browning or chewiness.

Most product manufacturers have their own proprietary blends, and cookbook authors typically vary in what they think is the ultimate flour blend. When experimenting, try cookbook authors' recommendations, then consider making your own tweaks by adding or subtracting ingredients and adjusting ratios to discover what works best for your particular recipes. Working with flour blends in gluten-free baking is both an art and science where constant experimentation is commonplace among expert chefs, cookbook authors, and home chefs alike.

What are some good flour blend formulas for wheat flour substitution?

Answers abound! But to recommend only a couple flour blends when there are a wide variety of quality options to choose from would be like having you test drive only two cars at the dealership among dozens of exceptional models. Your experience would be limited. So, embrace a journey of gluten-free flour blend discovery!

To begin experimenting with wheat flour substitutions at home, consult gluten-free cookbooks for an array of different gluten-free flour blends. You'll find many variations that are different from one another and many that are similar. You will often find white rice flour, tapioca flour, and potato starch in a blend, while others will capitalize on other flour combinations, some of which feature the rising star sorghum flour. Even quinoa flour, amaranth flour, sweet white rice flour, soy flour, and teff flour are being used in flour blends.

The flour blends you'll find in cookbooks have been tested and approved by the cookbook authors in their recipes, but don't be bashful in tweaking their ratios and flours to find the formula that suits your recipe needs best. Ask members of your local gluten-free support group about what blends they like and have found successful. Browse the Internet for options. If you like to bake from scratch, take on the search of a flour blend you will use regularly with a sense of adventure. Try many and have fun! Also, use the flour combinations you discover as guidelines for creating your own signature all-purpose flour blend. Consider making the flour blends in big batches so that they are at the ready for many of your baking needs. Store them well and use as you would use all-purpose flour.

Reality check: Remember that not all gluten-free recipes are created equal. While one flour blend will work well for one recipe another flour blend will not work as well for the same recipe. You've left the world of using just one flour (general all-purpose wheat flour) and have entered the realm of one size does not fit all. The gluten-free flour blend is like architecture, you have many materials at your disposal to build a quality structure and flavor in your baked goods. You simply have to find the materials that work best and that your palate enjoys most.

Why are certain gluten-free baked goods often dry and crumbly?

Gluten-free recipe development continues to improve by leaps and bounds, and as experimentation and recipes have become more advanced, two different camps on baking have arisen—one that suffers from dry and crumbly goods, and one that boasts moistness and chewiness. Whether a baked good is premade and sold in a package at a store or bakery, made at home from a mix, or made from scratch using a recipe, it will reside in one of these two camps. If your experiences continue to be disappointing, you simply have not found the right products or recipes yet—gluten-free baked goods don't have to be sub par.

There are numerous reasons why certain gluten-free baked goods such as bread, cookies, and muffins lack moisture and fall apart at the mere touch of your hands. The answer lies in the question: Where's the *gluten-free* glue and what kind of gluten-free glue is it?

When moistened, wheat-gluten takes on a glue-like consistency that binds ingredients together and provides structure for baked goods so they don't become dry and fall apart. Plus, gluten is essential to create "air pockets" in the baked good that helps produce that "spongy" quality. Remove the gluten, and you remove the glue and structure in a baked good. In gluten-free baking, the challenge is to replace the gluten with gluten-free glue. There are many ways to create gluten-free glue beyond adding xanthan gum. So, what could be the problem? Some possibilities could include:

- Using one gluten-free flour such as white rice flour (low protein) to replace the wheat flour, a practice often found in beginning baking experiments at home. It is rare in store-bought products and recent cookbooks.
- The flour blend utilizes just the white flours and starches that are low in protein and lack stickiness when moistened.
- Liquid, fat, or sweetening ingredients in proportion to the flour blend are not optimal and need reformulating.

Why do gluten-free baked goods often taste different from wheat-baked goods?

Certified master baker and gluten-free baking expert Richard Coppedge Jr. of The Culinary Institute of America in Hyde Park, New York provides insight on this one. Many gluten-free baked goods are made with a large amount of starchy flours, which include potato starch and tapioca starch made from root vegetables. By nature, these ingredients do not have much flavor, particularly after they are processed. And when potato starch and tapioca starch comprise two-thirds or more of the flour blend in a baked product, this ratio naturally contributes to the lack of flavor in the end product. Grain flours such as wheat naturally have more flavor, which is why traditional wheat-baked goods taste and smell so good!

The starches in gluten-free baking are primarily used as agents, meaning they serve a certain purpose for the baked good, either to bring weight and chewiness, or to make the product more airy and promote browning. They are not used for flavor, nor are they used to promote nutritional value. This is why many gluten-free breads become more palatable when toasted. The toasting helps caramelize the starch and boost the flavor. And oftentimes to compensate for the lack of flavor due to the root starches, gluten-free bakers will use sugar in excess.

Luckily, more gluten-free baked goods and recipes are now relying less on the large amount of starches in the flour blend and are incorporating more of the higher-protein, higher-flavor gluten-free flours into the blend, which will naturally improve the flavor. You'll notice that baked goods that rely more on the grain and seed flours such as sorghum, amaranth, quinoa, teff, corn, and rice have a better flavor and are often closer to capturing the flavor of a wheat-based product.

What improves the texture of gluten-free baked goods?

Many gluten-free baked goods can be described as crumbly, dry, dense, and brick-like. Baked goods with this description often have their roots in poorly developed recipes or pioneering experiments on the home front. But gluten-free nirvana does exist! Some of the most wonderfully delicious, well-structured baked goods you will ever taste happen to be gluten-free, developed by pioneering individuals and companies who have found out how to manipulate the ingredients to produce delicious, authentic baked goods.

While most gluten-free baked goods use xanthan gum or guar gum in the recipe to help bind the ingredients together and provide structure, recipes that use gums can still be terribly lacking in texture. So, what could be the larger issue at hand?

This is not a cookbook, and you're encouraged to consult some of the most *recently* published cookbooks on the topic—recipe development gets better every year. But a variety of factors can contribute to poor texture and oftentimes the answer is first found in the flour. The flours used in a recipe are critical. If you use just rice flour or a starch, you will have a texture problem, guaranteed. A combination of gluten-free flours works better together, and the kinds of flours used and their ratios are even more important because they each have certain baking powers. The older flour blend formulas used white rice flour, potato starch, and tapioca starch, which often produce a texture problem because simply there isn't enough protein in those flours. Recently, more baking experts are advising that gluten-free flour blends need to have higher protein content to improve structure and to augment the binding action that gums provide. Today, it's becoming more common to find flour blends using higher protein flours such as sorghum flour, teff flour, quinoa flour, amaranth flour, and even bean flours. So the best thing you can do to improve the texture of your gluten-free baked goods is to add a flour high in protein.

What improves moisture content of gluten-free baked goods?

Again, a wide array of factors can influence the moisture level of a gluten-free baked good. And naturally, the moisture level of a baked product is a key to its texture. If the baked good lacks moisture, poor texture will follow. If the moisture level is good, the baked good will hold together better and just have a nicer feel in your mouth. Many of the latest gluten-free cookbooks have recipes that can help steer you clear of moisture-deprived baking, but it's interesting to watch a sweet evolution taking place as more cookbook authors, bakers, and chefs are taking another look at sugar and its moisture holding properties.

The days of strictly using white granulated sugar in recipes are numbered—more and more bakers are looking to other sugars and natural sweeteners that hold in moisture. For example, sugars that have more color are less refined and stickier, which can be a good thing for making cookies. The stickiness in moisture-holding sweeteners can help with the binding factor of ingredients in addition to the protein in your flour blend. Today, in lieu of traditional white sugar, more attention is being given to sweeteners such as Agave nectar, honey, gluten-free brown rice syrup, molasses, pure brown cane sugar crystals, and turbinado sugar.

Also, the fats used in a recipe have an impact on the moisture and chewy factor of a baked good. Healthy vegetable oils such as safflower oil have moisture-holding properties and are becoming more widely used in lieu of butter.

Tip: Slightly undercooking your cookies can help hold in moisture.

Are gums required for gluten-free baking?

It's extremely common to find xanthan gum and guar gum used in gluten-free products and they are regularly called for in gluten-free cookbook recipes, so it's easy to assume that you can't make gluten-free baked goods *without* them. But can you? The answer is yes, although many in the gluten-free baking world would disagree.

The challenge in baking gluten-free without xanthan gum or guar gum boils down to using other ingredients that work well together to replicate the binding and fluffy quality of gluten-baked goods. Gluten is sticky, so you need ingredients that are sticky, bind flours together well, contribute moisture, and add structure all at the same time. This task can be a challenging one. But pastry chefs continue to experiment. Cindy Gawel, a vegan pastry chef based in Denver, Colorado who specializes in made-to-order gluten-free baked goods and confections, does not use gums in her baking. She looks for all natural ingredients that are sticky in and of themselves. For example, she says that amaranth flour and sweet white rice flour work well together in a flour blend to help create the stickiness produced by gluten in wheat flour. She also encourages the use of sticky, moisture-holding sweeteners like agave nectar or turbinado sugar to help create a sticky, binding-effect.

Xanthan gum and guar gum continue to be primary ingredients for gluten-free baking. But as chefs, cookbook authors, and consumers become more familiar with the art of gluten-free baking and continue to explore which ingredients and flours work well together to mimic gluten, there may be less reliance on xanthan gum and guar gum in the future.

What are some easy recipe substitutions to make a traditional recipe gluten-free?

Once you get the hang of your gluten-free diet, you become evermore savvy in the ways of creative recipe substitutions. Your thinking naturally adopts a "what if" approach and you'll experiment with different gluten-free ingredients in your favorite recipes. There are no wrong answers, just opportunities to explore and play with tradition! Don't hold back. Experimentation is a part of the gluten-free life … always. You'll often be delightfully surprised with what you come up with.

But in the beginning, the creative gluten-free substitution wheels aren't always as well-oiled. The following examples illustrate some simplistic approaches to making traditional foods gluten-free. Making baked items such as breads, cookies, and cakes are more advanced and require even more experimentation, using different flour blends to see what works best and tweaking a recipe's chemistry.

- Meatloaf or meatballs: Replace bread crumbs with your own freshly made bread crumbs using slices of toasted gluten-free bread, crumbled gluten-free crackers, or rice.

- Noodles: Substitute gluten-free rice noodles when traditional egg noodles are called for in a recipe.
- Barbecued meats: Substitute gluten-free barbecue sauce for regular sauce.
- Italian pasta dishes: Replace traditional wheat pasta with gluten-free Italian-style pasta.
- Gravies: Instead of wheat flour, thicken with corn starch, potato starch, arrowroot starch, or rice flour. Consult cookbooks for guidelines on using the ingredients properly.
- Macaroni and cheese: Replace traditional wheat elbow macaroni with gluten-free elbow macaroni and substitute finely ground rice flour for any small amount of wheat flour the recipe calls for to thicken the cheese sauce.
- Cheesecake: Choose recipes for cream cheese filling that don't call for flour to raise the filling. Be creative with replacing the graham cracker crust—try gluten-free biscotti cookie crumbs, gluten-free crumbled cookies, or hazelnut meal for example.
- Asian dishes: Where soy sauce is the only forbidden ingredient, simply substitute wheat-free soy sauce.
- Small amounts of wheat flour: For recipes that call for one to three tablespoons or so of all-purpose flour such as goulashes, stroganoff, creamed corn, or soufflés, experiment with a gluten-free cup-for-cup substitution flour blend.
- Leave it out: Have you often wondered why a small amount of flour is included in a recipe and question if it really makes all that much difference? In these cases, simply leave it out!
- Go crust-free! Many pies can be enjoyed without making the crust, thus making them deliciously gluten-free. Honestly, how many people do you know eat the pumpkin pie just for the custard anyway?

What are some gluten-free cookbooks?

Bette Hagman, otherwise fondly known as The Gluten-Free Gourmet, is one of the pioneering authors and gluten-free recipe developers. Since Hagman authored her first authoritative and comprehensive recipe book on the subject in 1990, *The Gluten-Free Gourmet: Living Well Without Wheat*, there has been a steady growth of gluten-free cookbooks. Now, the gluten-free cookbook market is proliferating, which is good news for a growing celiac and gluten-intolerant population with varying cooking and baking interests and tastes.

As more publishers recruit experts to develop gluten-free cookbooks, following is a mere slice of what's available to get you started in either building your personal library of many books or simply finding one to get you by if you don't spend much time in the kitchen.

Annalise G. Roberts
  Gluten-Free Baking Classics
Bette Hagman
  The Gluten-Free Gourmet Cooks Comfort Foods: Creating Old Favorites with the New Flours
  The Gluten-Free Gourmet Bakes Bread: More Than 200 Wheat-Free Recipes
  The Gluten-Free Gourmet Cooks Fast and Healthy: Wheat-Free Recipes with Less Fuss and Less Fat
  The Gluten-Free Gourmet Cooks Fast and Healthy
  The Gluten-Free Gourmet Makes Dessert
  The Gluten-Free Gourmet, Second Edition: Living Well Without Wheat
Carol Fenster
  Gluten-Free 101
  Cooking Free

Wheat-Free Recipes & Menus

Gluten-Free Quick and Easy: From Prep to Plate Without the Fuss

1000 Gluten-Free Recipes (To be released 2008)

Connie Sarros

Wheat-Free Gluten-Free Cookbook for Kids & Busy Adults

Wheat-Free Gluten-Free Reduced Calorie Cookbook

Wheat-Free, Gluten-Free Dessert Book

Darina Allen and Rosemary Kearney

Healthy Gluten-Free Cooking: 150 Recipes for Food Lovers

Donna Washburn & Heather Butt

Complete Gluten-Free Cookbook:150 Gluten-Free, Lactose-Free Recipes, Many With Egg-Free Variations

The Best Gluten-Free Family Cookbook

Jacqueline Mallorca

The Wheat-Free Cook: Gluten-Free Recipes for Everyone

Rebecca Reilly

Gluten-Free Baking: More Than 125 Recipes Delectable Sweet and Savory Baked Goods

Richard Coppedge

Gluten-Free Baking with The Culinary Institute of America (To be released 2008)

Rick Marx and Nancy Maar

The Everything Gluten-Free Cookbook: 300 Appetizing Recipes Tailored To Your Needs!

And if you want an authoritative cookbook on the world of grains—including the primary gluten-free grains—the 2007 James Beard Foundation awarding-winning cookbook *Whole Grains Everyday Every Way* by Lorna Sass features an in-depth look at all of these grains, complete with recipes.

What are some websites where you can find gluten-free recipes?

A world of online gluten-free recipe sites awaits you. Plus, finding gluten-free recipes online can take you to companies and individuals who provide recipes of different countries' native cuisines and foods you may have never thought to try.

When searching on the net you can virtually stumble upon countless avenues to gluten-free recipes, some of which are from individually sponsored sites, companies, community support groups, online recipe blogs, and swaps. To get you started, some Web sites with an ample library of recipes include:

www.glutenfree.com
www.bestglutenfreerecipes.com
www.recipezaar.com
www.livingwithout.com

Tips for finding gluten-free recipes online include visiting:
- Food company Web sites that sell gluten-free flours and grains such as www.bobsredmill.com. They have a large library of recipes featuring their ingredients.
- Web sites operated by gluten-free cookbook authors
- Your local celiac or community support group chapter may have recipes posted on their site.
- Go to culinary magazine websites and type gluten-free recipes into their search bar.
- Web sites operated by natural foods markets
- Or simply type "gluten-free recipes" into your favorite search engine and peruse what comes up.

Are some pieces of equipment better than others for gluten-free baking?

As you begin the the process of cleaning your kitchen to make it gluten-free, you may find the need to replace some equipment because it didn't pass the test for eliminating cross-contamination (Chapter Five). Or if you plan to make gluten-free baking a regular aspect of your life, you may want to consider buying some new equipment just to start fresh. But if you wonder if there are better pieces of equipment than others for your gluten-free baking pursuits, you've asked the right question. Not all types of equipment are best suited for the gluten-free baking or cooking challenge and a piece's performance properties can be quite important when it comes to the quirky nuances of gluten-free baking in particular.

Below are a few tips to get you started, but you will find that gluten-free cookbook authors are the experts to consult on this topic. You'll find helpful tips and hints in their cookbooks based on their experience with recipes they've developed.

Gluten-free baking is a batter-focused art and you'll find most gluten-free cake and bread batters will be sticky. This calls for nonstick baking equipment that will release your baked goods easily. Also, look for equipment that has hygienic food grade silicone because it won't latch onto odors and flavors. Teflon is a natural choice for nonstick. But cookbook author Carol Fenster urges you to stick to the grey nonstick cookware, not the fancy black nonstick variety. Avoiding glass and metal bakeware is also recommended by some experts also.

In lieu of nonstick Teflon, consider purchasing loaf pans made from a cardboard-like material with "waxy" walls inside. These pans are extremely convenient and are perfect for storing your baked goods in the freezer, and they are fantastic for making baked goods as gifts. Flexible silicon baking molds also come highly recommended.

And if you are in the market for a bread machine, look for models that have gluten-free bread baking settings.

Can a bread machine make gluten-free bread?

If you've become attached to working with bread machines prior to going gluten-free and you'd like to keep using your current model, or if you're in search of just the perfect model for gluten-free baking, there's good news and there's bad news.

The bad news

Nearly all bread machines are designed for gluten-based breads, not gluten-free breads. Using a traditional bread machine to make gluten-free bread is like trying to boil pasta in the microwave. It can be done, but not without a lot of babysitting, finagling of directions, asking the machine to do things differently from what it was designed to do, and producing different results. And while bread machines are supposed to be time saving, you'll find that making a gluten-free bread in a bread machine doesn't necessarily save time off the clock. First, bread machines are designed for two risings. Many gluten-free yeast breads require only one rise. And if you don't have a machine where you can control the cycles so you can bypass the second cycle, you'll waste time watching over it. Also, machines with the ability to control the cycles typically cost more.

The good news

Consult gluten-free baking books and you'll find some savvy tricks to outsmart the machine and possibly be on your way to enjoying a good gluten-free loaf. For example, because gluten-free bread batter is sticky and dense, many say a heavy paddle will work best. And despite having a nonstick bucket, still augment with some spray or butter to prevent a not-so-desirable release. Tips can be found to help you with this gluten-free baking challenge in a traditional bread machine if you are set on using one. Carol Fenster has an arsenal of tips on how to outsmart the traditional bread machine in her book *Gluten-Free 101, Easy, Basic Dishes Without Wheat* and Ener-G Foods provides some advice on their website, www.ener-g.com.

Manufacturers are now taking notice of the need to design their new models with gluten-free bread settings, and more models are bound to appear on store shelves in the future. Currently, Cuisinart has a machine with a gluten-free setting, as does the Breadman TR875 2-Pound Stainless Steel Breadmaker.

Chapter 14

FAMILY AND CHILDREN: WHAT THEY NEED TO KNOW

- What if you are the only one in the house who must eat gluten-free?
- Should your family eat gluten-free too?
- How can your family be supportive of you living gluten-free?
- Should all members of the household or family be tested for celiac disease?
- How can you help convince your immediate family members they should get tested?
- What are some tactics for dealing with the holidays?
- What are some strategies for family menu planning?
- How can you best inform school staff about your child's dietary needs?
- What are some gluten-free snack suggestions for children?
- How can you explain to your small child that *you* can't eat foods with wheat gluten?
- How can you explain to your child that *they* can no longer eat foods with wheat and gluten?
- How can a young child eat gluten-free at school?
- How can your child remain vigilant at school and beat peer pressure?

What if you are the only one in the house who must eat gluten-free?

Even if you are the only gluten-free pioneer in the household, the gluten-free lifestyle becomes a family adventure. Unlike medical or health conditions that require medications or other lifestyle adjustments, celiac disease and nonceliac gluten-intolerance revolve around one common thing—food—which affects everyone you live with.

Living the gluten-free lifestyle is unavoidably high maintenance, particularly at first, and in order to live safely as well as efficiently, the whole family needs to become just as knowledgeable about the foods you can and cannot eat as if they had to follow the diet themselves. All family members old enough to grocery shop need to learn what gluten is, where it is found, and how to avoid it (Chapter Three). Shopping, cooking, and cleaning are often shared responsibilities, and your family will inevitably become involved in buying gluten-free foods for you, avoiding foods with gluten, reading ingredient labels, and being aware of and avoiding cross-contamination issues at home. This shared knowledge among the family will be particularly helpful for times when you are sick and need help with the shopping and cooking, or when taking family vacations, throwing surprise birthday parties, entertaining, looking after you if you're in the hospital, and so forth.

By educating everyone in the house about the gluten-free lifestyle, you will feel supported and not so alone. In fact, the whole family can share in the joy of helping you live the lifestyle as well as experience the pleasures of eating gluten-free with you. Living gluten-free is a family affair and does not need to be undertaken alone.

Should your family eat gluten-free too?

Living a strict gluten-free lifestyle can be limiting and expensive, and there is no reason for the entire family to do it if it's not absolutely necessary. However, there are many benefits if your family eats gluten-free with you at home. When the whole family eats mostly gluten-free with you, menu planning, avoiding cross-contact, managing cravings, and even budget control can be easier. Why buy two kinds of pasta when the gluten-free version will make everyone happy?

Even with the abundance of gluten-free foods available, transitioning into the gluten-free lifestyle is challenging at first. If your family could live gluten-free with you for at least the first month, it would be a wonderful show of support and provide encouragement as you move through this phase. Plus, by following a gluten-free diet with you for a period of time, it's possible that some family members may discover that symptoms they once struggled with or took for granted may subside and as a result more members of the family may choose to eat gluten-free as well. If you have celiac disease or gluten-intolerance it's possible that other blood relatives in your household could have the celiac gene also. And even though chances are higher for other members having the condition, there is no statistic that explains this probability or risk.

But if you are the only one who must eat gluten-free and your family is resistant to going completely gluten-free with you, perhaps they could eat gluten-free with you every other week or once a month. It's a wonderful way to introduce them to new products, unique ingredients, and recipes you've discovered on your journey. In fact, a gluten-free diet offers a multitude of ingredients, recipes, and products that the entire family can enjoy and nutritionally benefit from.

Bottom Line: It's important that your family learn and practice the diet with you at least during your transition period to show support, provide encouragement, and help everyone learn about the diet so they can support you properly when needed.

How can your family be supportive of you living gluten-free?

Living gluten-free can be isolating if you feel you're the only one who knows what you go through on a daily basis. Try to educate your friends and family about a gluten-free diet because the more they know, the more they can help support you.

Family members need to know enough about the diet to help prepare meals, shop, and prepare for traveling. It's your job to educate them. Make sure they know what gluten is, where it's found, and how to avoid it. Consider taking a class and ask your spouse, parent, or friend to attend with you. While they may never become an expert (like you must), simply making the effort to understand the gluten-free lifestyle will be helpful and comforting to you.

But there are times when sensitivity should be practiced also. Baking a huge batch of your favorite wheat-based fudge brownies or chocolate chip cookies in front of you, particularly in the transitional weeks of going gluten-free, is not the most supportive thing your family can do.

They can support you by being open to new tastes, ingredients, recipes, and products that you bring home or experiment with. Saying "Yuck! You'll never get me to try that," is not being supportive and understanding. Encourage experimentation!

Invite family and friends over for a gluten-free food night where you have a variety of foods prepared from scratch as well as packaged products they can taste. This is a fun way to help educate family and friends about the diet. Create gluten-free question games to spice up the event, making it educational and memorable.

Should all members of the household or family be tested for celiac disease?

The answer is yes if any of the following are true: If you have been tested and diagnosed positive for celiac disease and therefore carry the genetic marker; if a close relative of the family has been tested and diagnosed positive; if anyone in the family has one or more of the chronic symptoms or complications associated with celiac disease; or if someone in the family has eliminated gluten from their diet and has come to believe that gluten is without question the reason behind their illness and discomfort.

When you're embarking upon a lifetime of following a gluten-free diet and it's known that the condition can be hereditary, it's highly recommended to know for certain who in your family has the condition. It's too serious to not know for sure who has it and who does not. When left undiagnosed, serious complications can occur. Conclusive evidence will provide an unbiased baseline for understanding long-term family care and strategizing the household's eating habits. It can also make you aware and prepared for the possibility that any new children could carry the gene and might develop the condition. Knowing who has celiac disease and who does not immediately eliminates guesswork regarding mysterious symptoms, streamlines shopping and menu planning, and can make everyone happy, healthy, and safe.

But be prepared for resistance! Not everyone in your immediate family is going to welcome the opportunity to get tested with open arms, and your efforts to nudge them lovingly into doing so may be difficult. Even though you may suspect a parent, sibling, or spouse has celiac disease, they may not be as concerned about it as you are and will not feel it's necessary enough to warrant the perceived hassle of a doctor's visit. But continue to encourage them because left undiagnosed, the condition could lead to long-term complications including disease, depression, and the inability to have children. Don't wait, and be persistent.

How can you help convince your immediate family members they should get tested?

If you've discovered you have celiac disease, it's natural to want to know who else in the family has the condition. If no one else in your household or immediate relatives have been screened for indicators of the disease, whether they exhibit symptoms or not, it's time to at least start talking about it. But it's an all too common complaint that family members are resistant to being tested for gluten-intolerance and celiac disease even though symptoms or family history strongly suggest they should be. Although reasons (or shall we say excuses!) abound for wanting to dodge the bullet, it's your role to push the envelope if you think it's necessary.

Of course, the thought of receiving a positive diagnosis is by no means appealing, but they must know definitively so that they can properly care for themselves. There are two crucial reasons to be tested:

Preventative maintenance

Celiac disease, if left unchecked, can lead to serious complications that can be life threatening. Of all reasons, this should be the most convincing!

In the name of children

If there are children in the household or if there are plans to have a family and one parent/spouse has been positively diagnosed, the other parent/spouse should be tested also. This is particularly important because it's establishing a family history that can be helpful for children, grandchildren, and future generations. With heredity being a link for this disease, it's selfish to refuse testing that can be used to help properly diagnose members now and provide helpful information for future members of the family tree.

What are some tactics for dealing with the holidays?

If there was ever a time of the year when your patience with gluten-free living will be tested, it's the holidays. While gluten-free recipes for holiday fare are widely available, gluten-free cooking and baking are not the most difficult aspects of the holidays. There are other, more important things to be concerned with to keep you safe and satisfied.

- Holiday parties are not the best time to play the gluten guessing game. Bring what you can eat and enjoy to the holiday party—what you bring may be the *only* thing you can eat, so a fruit plate may not fit the bill.
- If you're traveling to see family, offer to bring a dish or two. Consider bringing a homemade gluten-free stuffing that can be baked in a separate casserole dish, or make a gluten-free bread. Share lists of ingredients you must avoid with your family so they will know what you cannot eat, and give them tips for avoiding cross-contact. After the trimmings have been served it is not the right time to ask if the same spoon used to serve the bread stuffing was used to serve you from the gluten-free potato casserole.
- Consider forwarding your family gluten-free recipes or offer to send or bring packages of gluten-free rice flour, tapioca flour, arrowroot starch, or cornstarch to act as replacements for things like the wheat in the gravy.
- If you dine out with family, your gluten-free option detection skills will be tested. Consider calling ahead to the restaurant to let them know what you'll need so they can make some gluten-free holiday fare suggestions prior to your arrival.
- When visiting family for just a few hours, consider eating before you go. Being satisfied upon arrival will help when you must pass the bowl of stuffing the other way and refuse dipping the

carrot stick in the mystery dip. And always remember, if in doubt, don't put it on your plate.

What are some strategies for family menu planning?

When cooking gluten-free in a household that is not, you have three basic choices: (1) Make your gluten-free meal separate from the other meals; (2) Make a meal that can be made gluten-free for you with one or two adjustments; (3) Or make a 100 percent gluten-free meal that the whole family can enjoy. A combination of these choices is usually the most realistic, but over time, making your meals separate or cooking two versions of the same meal can become time consuming, expensive, and exasperating. Regularly making gluten-free meals is probably the best option, but you must find a way to make it enjoyable for the whole family.

Sit down with your family and draft a list of your favorite foods and recipes for breakfast, lunch, and dinner. Separate the foods that are naturally gluten-free from the ones that are not. Take the non-gluten-free recipe favorites and begin converting them to delicious gluten-free versions. Pasta recipes such as spaghetti, lasagna, and macaroni and cheese will be easy to convert using the many brands of packaged gluten-free pastas to choose from.

Converting other recipes such as pizza, fried chicken, meatloaf, and chicken parmesan using gluten-free flours and products will be more challenging, but don't think you can't do it. Isolate the gluten in the recipe and research gluten-free cookbooks on how to use alternative ingredients.

With gluten-free breads, muffins, cakes, crusts, pancakes, pasta, etc., even if they're resistant, your family should try what you eat at least once. Chances are they will often be just as happy as you are and you can save time and money in the long run by buying gluten-free products for the whole family.

Find happy mediums in planning meals throughout the week. Consider designating certain nights as gluten-friendly for the family, then cook your own gluten-free meal on those days. Experiment with different menus and habits to find a routine that makes all of you happy and healthy.

How can you best inform school staff about your child's dietary needs?

Regardless of the level of celiac awareness in your child's school, you must take the initiative to let the staff know your child cannot have gluten under any circumstances. Making a few phone calls and in-person visits are always wise so that you can develop a relationship with the individuals who work closely with your child, and they will feel comfortable calling you if they have questions. This includes the principal, teachers, nurse, and cafeteria manager. It's always best to augment verbal communication with written reference lists, tips, and contact information. Craft a letter or email to school personnel who need to know and be sensitive to your child's needs. Even if your child is not celiac, but gluten-intolerant, the same strict measures apply.

A sample letter to use as a guide follows:

> My child, (insert name), has celiac disease (or is gluten-intolerant). This is a serious digestive disorder where he/she cannot eat foods or come into contact with materials that contain gluten. Gluten is a protein found in wheat, barley, and rye. Oats must also be avoided. If he/she eats or touches anything with gluten, he/she will get extremely sick. Snacks, cookies, cupcakes, cakes, bread, cereal, and many other foods have gluten in them. Also, classroom materials that must be avoided include playdough because of probable wheat in the dough and possibly paints and crayons that contain gluten.

When there is snack time or special food activities in class, my child can eat fresh fruits and vegetables, plain popcorn, etc. (Fill in accordingly). With advance notice of a classmate's in-class birthday celebration, I can have my child bring his/her own gluten-free treat to enjoy with the class.

For easy reference, please find attached a list of common foods and materials that my child must avoid, as well as gluten-free snack suggestions the whole class might like.

I understand that you may have some questions and please don't hesitate to call me to discuss. Thank you very much for your cooperation and monitoring the situation. I look forward to working with you.

What are some gluten-free snack suggestions for children?

For children, snacking can be the highlight of their day. Not only do they look forward to it, snacks can be healthy energy boosters and mood enhancers. Nothing beats a snack that tastes great, satisfies in-between meal hunger pangs, and is nutritious at the same time. However, thinking up creative gluten-free snacks that children actually enjoy can be a daunting task. While fresh fruits and vegetables are fantastic and gluten-free packaged snacks such as cookies can fit the bill for awhile, many parents will end up scratching their heads for other options.

Women's and parent's magazines can be great sources for ideas—they've done the market research and often feature "kid's favorites" snack ideas. You can also try typing things like "Top 10 Healthy Snacks for Children" into your favorite search engine and see what you can find. This exercise can help you think outside of the box and come up with some really innovative and delicious snack ideas that are gluten-free.

Consider the following gluten-free snack transformations:

- An Old Favorite
  - Rice Krispie treats can be made with gluten-free rice puff cereal and gluten-free marshmallows. Transform the traditional recipe with your gluten-free ingredients.
- Mini-Pizzas
  - Use rice cakes, gluten-free crackers, or slices of gluten-free bread for "crust." Pile on various toppings and cheese and melt in the toaster oven.
- Nut Butter Balls
  - Use peanut or almond butter and dried fruit such as raisins or cherries, combine the butter with a bit of gluten-free milk powder and honey, then roll it into balls. Coat the balls with crumbled up gluten-free cookies.
- Mini-Muffins
  - Bake a batch of mini-muffins using a gluten-free baking mix. Add gluten-free chocolate chips to the batter.
- Trail Mix
  - Combine gluten-free cereal shapes with raisins, chocolate chips, peanuts, and gluten-free pretzels.
- Freeze It
  - Make frozen pudding pops using gluten-free pudding and molds.

How can you explain to your small child that *you* can't eat foods with wheat gluten?

For parents who discover their gluten-intolerance later in life, your children will inevitably want to know why you can't eat the same things. Rather than respond with something like "What you eat makes me sick," which could translate inappropriately to a young mind and possibly produce fear and confusion, a better approach is a positive statement such as: "You are able to eat foods with wheat flour because your tummy doesn't get upset. I don't have the same ability you do, but there are many other good foods I can eat that don't contain wheat." Reinforce your explanation with something gluten-free that your child can taste. If your child is more mature and inquisitive, you should be more open with your symptoms so they can be more supportive of you and help you where they can.

How can you explain to your child that *they* can no longer eat foods with wheat and gluten?

Telling a child they can no longer eat the foods they enjoy is no easy task for any parent. The child's age, their ability to comprehend language and concepts, and how accustomed they are to eating gluten-based foods will have an impact on how well your explanation and actions are received. The child's doctor can play an important role in delivering the news too, but you have the challenge of holding the line on the home front.

Given a scenario where the child is old enough to understand your words and actions, following are some points to keep in mind:

- Let your child know that their health is your main priority and the decisions you make are in the name of their well-being; you're not being "mean."
- Let them know they are not alone and that many children or even their own family members are not able to eat foods with wheat and gluten.
- While you don't want to scare them, it's critical to let them know how important it is that they avoid the foods that are not good for them. For them, avoiding wheat and gluten is as important as a child who must avoid peanuts due to a severe allergy.

- Even if your child has celiac disease, it's important that they don't feel as if something is wrong with them. Any way you can make them proud and feel special for eating gluten-free foods will be beneficial in the long-term.
- Let them know they are not alone. And to make them feel better, you are simply going to replace certain foods like cookies and pasta with other gluten-free cookies and pasta to enjoy. They are made with different ingredients that won't make their tummy ache. These foods have the power to make them feel better. These foods are your friends. They not only taste good, they will make you healthier.

How can a young child eat gluten-free at school?

For young people of any age with celiac disease or gluten-intolerance, school can be full of potential gluten pitfalls, as well as temptations, if they're not coached on how to avoid gluten and given the tools they need to succeed.

As if parents didn't have enough to think and worry about when their children attend school, the following list provides ideas to think about as well as processes to implement for any parent with school age, gluten-intolerant children.

- Cafeteria lunches will be hit or miss, but more often than not they will have gluten in one or more menu items on any given day. Provide balanced and nutritious gluten-free lunches for a child to take daily, as well as snacks to eat during breaks.
- Consult the principal and cafeteria manager on which foods are regularly gluten-free and which foods to avoid. Also, discuss potential cross-contact issues to avoid. Let them know who your child is so they can watch out for them.

- Let every applicable teacher know that your child must avoid gluten when food is brought into the classroom.
- For preschools, playdough must be off-limits for your child and the teacher must know.
- Regardless of age, children may be tempted into consuming foods containing gluten that are offered to them by others—and the foods probably aren't offered out of malice, but of the child wanting to be polite and share or through sheer misunderstanding of the disease. Make sure your child understands the importance of not consuming gluten, and it's probably best to have a teacher watch a young child and make sure he or she does not eat anything dangerous.
- Teach your child how to read ingredient labels and to recognize foods with gluten. They must become vigilant and watch out for hidden gluten.
- Consulting with staff and advance planning will be necessary each time a field trip or sporting event away from school takes place.
- Vending machines should be off-limits unless certain foods have been confirmed gluten-free.
- Every young person needs to be prepared to know how to explain their gluten-intolerance and what they must avoid to anyone when the need arises.

How can your child remain vigilant at school and beat peer pressure?

Gluten-free living is challenging for adults, and it can be double the challenge for young people. No child wants to feel sick, and knowing what will make them feel ill and how to avoid it will help them stay healthy. But expecting children of any age to adhere to the strict guidelines of a gluten-free diet, particularly when away from home, is asking them to rise to a level of maturity, discipline, and fortitude that many other children do not have to take on. But youngsters are smart and adaptable. As it's often easier for young people to learn foreign languages than adults, learning the ins and outs of gluten-free living at a young age can be done, but tools and know-how are the key.

- Give your child a list of foods and brand name products they have to avoid, and make sure they keep the list with them at all times. They will have to learn how to read labels as an adult would when they are on their own buying packaged foods.
- Have your child take part in making their bag lunch. Let them help bake their gluten-free cookies, make snacks, and mix batter. When children have a personal investment in their food and like what they make, they'll be less likely to give into gluten temptation at school or trade for something that can be harmful to them. Another child will not know if something is forbidden or not.
- Except for fruits and vegetables, children need to say no to food that is offered to them by others, including candy. But if they have their own gluten-free food to enjoy, they will be protective of it and saying no won't be as difficult.
- When your child visits friends, the parents need to know the dietary restrictions to help keep your child safe. Slumber parties, birthday parties, and backyard fiestas can be difficult times for a child, and gluten-free options need to be available so they don't feel excluded or different.
- When teenagers are in a rebellious stage, sticking to the diet may be one of the things they rebel against. Emphasize to your children that it's cool to stay healthy and safe.
- Just like adults, children have cravings too. They will need healthy gluten-free snacks on hand to fight the munchies.

Chapter 15

FRIENDS, SOCIAL EVENTS, AND WORK: TIPS FOR HOLDING THE LINE

- When a friend invites you over for a meal, how do you eat gluten-free?
- How can you educate your host/hostess about ingredients you can't eat?
- How do you avoid gluten at important sit-down affairs?
- What are some tips for attending potlucks and parties?
- What are some strategies for attending social events?
- How do you find out about all ingredients used in a dish prepared by someone else?
- How do you navigate around possible cross-contact issues in a dish prepared by someone else?
- What should you do about wedding and birthday cake?
- What are suggestions for gluten-free foods and snacks for backpacking and camping trips?
- Can you eat gluten-free at the movies, amusement parks, and sporting events?
- Should you let your boss and coworkers know about your gluten-intolerance?
- How do you avoid cross-contact with gluten at work?
- How can you best handle business meetings at restaurants?
- What are some gluten-free snack suggestions for the office?

When a friend invites you over for a meal, how do you eat gluten-free?

Once you begin living gluten-free, the first dinner party invite can be a bit tricky or slightly uncomfortable if not handled with care. While it's natural to be grateful for whatever your host serves you, when you're gluten-intolerant you have no choice but to let them know what you can and cannot eat before they begin shopping and preparing a meal for you.

From an etiquette perspective this can feel awkward, particularly if you're not all that close with the host. But the worst thing you can do is not say anything and cross your fingers that you will be able to eat what they prepare. You'll run the risk of getting sick or being embarrassed when you let your host know you can't eat what they may have spent hours making. Avoid this unpleasant scenario with the following tips for handling an invitation with poise.

- When you receive an invitation to dinner, be proactive from the start. First, let your host know how thankful you are, but that you can't eat wheat and gluten and your dietary needs can be quite challenging. This may be unfamiliar territory for your host and they will likely have several questions. Offer to email a list of the most common ingredients that you must avoid as a primer for your host when designing their menu and shopping list.
- Offer to bring gluten-free alternatives such as salad dressing, dinner rolls, or even wheat-free soy sauce if a stir-fry is planned. Politely try to find out all ingredients being used before you eat, and best case scenario, before the dinner is even made. Questions up front will eliminate apologies later.
- Offer to bring a gluten-free dessert as a gesture of appreciation and to take the stress off your host for this often tricky portion of the meal.

How can you educate your host/hostess about ingredients you can't eat?

Eating a gluten-free meal at someone's house can be challenging, particularly if they don't know a gluten-free diet protocol. However, if you don't share information with your host about your dietary needs, uncomfortable situations are bound to occur. You'll get used to providing verbal dissertations on what you can and can't eat, but frankly, you'll get tired of giving the spiel over and over again, particularly if your lifestyle involves a great deal of social engagements.

While each situation is different and will call for a personalized approach, it can be worthwhile to have a ready-made mini-reference handout you've created for this type of situation. When the host asks you what you can and cannot eat, you can give them a brief primer on the diet but also offer to send them your handout when you feel it's appropriate and not impolite to do so. In fact, the host may be appreciative of the help. This handout will be handy for your hosts' menu planning whether they are friends, family or acquaintances.

When designing your handout, consider including the following:

- A simple definition of gluten and some common names for wheat and gluten.
- A list of common foods where gluten is found. For example, be sure to mention pasta as a culprit for lunch or dinner, and cereal, toast, and pancakes for breakfast.
- Common ingredients found in the refrigerator and cupboard where hidden gluten can be found (i.e. soy sauce, prepared meats, marinades, and ice cream).
- Recommendations for certain gluten-free versions of foods that can be found at a nearby store.
- Offer to bring a dish or specific ingredient.

- A list of gluten-free recipe websites you recommend, and foods or recipes you enjoy.
- A note about cross-contamination and how to avoid it. Include a list of quick and polite reminders, such as leaving off the croutons from the salad.
- A warm note of appreciation at the end for taking the time to accommodate your dietary needs. Let them know they can call you should they have questions.
- Make the handout look pretty so that it's fun to read and softens the hard news.

How do you avoid gluten at important sit-down affairs?

When you have no control over what is being served at a large catered affair like a wedding, an annual awards dinner or charity event, you must approach the event with low expectations and know that ingredient disclosure will probably not be as readily available as it can be in restaurants. Catered meals are ordered well in advance, are often prepared off-site, and brought to the venue in warming ovens. The chef or catering company owner may not be at the event to ask questions about ingredients, and the servers may not know. You might be at the mercy of your educated guess-work.

Before you sit down for a preplated meal, try to ask a server as soon as you can what is being served. This way you can get an idea if the main course will have gluten and if so, you can try to request basic adjustments before your plate is served. Given enough lead time, the catering staff may be able to put something special together for you. But in any case, try to avoid waiting to see what is delivered to your table. Instead, be proactive in the beginning. Special requests made after the meal is served can lead to numerous delays with your meal, or worse, you could go hungry.

If you know the host or organizer of the event, try to arrange a special meal days in advance. With buffets, gluten-free options are usually limited and you'll have to do your best to choose the items you believe will be safe. Bottom line: Eating ahead before you attend a catered affair is always a good rule if you don't want to take any chances.

What are some tips for attending potlucks and parties?

Potlucks and parties are famous for having a smorgasbord of foods, very few of which are gluten-free. But you don't have to go hungry! These gatherings are easily manageable because you can be in control and bring something you've made to share with the group. But plan on what you bring to be the only thing you can eat—and if there are other options, you can be pleasantly surprised.

If you don't bring your own food, you'll find yourself playing the gluten guessing game with each dish down the line. Navigate your way through the foods as you would the deli section of the grocery store (Chapter Eight). You will be able to eliminate certain dishes right away because of the visible gluten. But you then have to watch out for the hidden gluten. These food fests are always full of risk, where each prepared food is a mystery dish. Decide how much investigative work you want to do, or simply eat the dish you brought.

If veggie sticks and fruit are not your idea of satisfying meal, think again about bringing your own food, eat before you go, or plan on eating after the event. And be prepared for gluten cravings to stimulate your appetite. These events will usually test your patience, but are great training grounds for building confidence in saying no to the foods that seem so tempting.

What are some strategies for attending social events?

Socializing and food go together like salt and pepper; it's rare that you find one without the other. And with food usually being a main attraction, it's often just as fun if not more so than the company and conversation. How many times have you gone to an event just to eat the food? Probably more often than you'd like to admit. But when you're living gluten-free, attending social events requires a shift in thinking and an adjustment of expectations. Unless they are gluten-free events, you probably won't find many safe foods. So, visiting with others will now take center stage and the food of the party takes a back seat.

However, when you want to find something you can eat, there are some navigation rules to keep in mind:

Social Event Rule Number #1: Have an idea ahead of time if there will be someone you can ask about mystery dishes. Asking questions at large catered affairs where the staff is invisible is usually more difficult than at parties hosted by friends or associates. If you know there won't be someone you can get accurate information from, you're on your own and you'll need to play it extra safe.

Social Event Rule #2: Change your thinking from attending the event for the food to just looking for something to snack on. Then, if you can't find anything to eat, your expectations were low from the beginning.

Social Event Rule #3: When looking at the spread, make the distinction between singular, raw unprocessed foods and foods that are processed or dishes with multiple ingredients. Use your gluten-detection skills (Chapter Three) to find what's safe and, worse come to worse, stick to the fruit and vegetable trays.

How do you find out about all ingredients used in a dish prepared by someone else?

If there is something you're just dying to try, but you don't know if it's gluten-free, you might be inclined to investigate further. If you know the host or guest who made the dish, you probably won't be bashful in asking about the ingredients. However, if you don't know who made the dish, you'll have a challenge on your hands. In this case it will be best not to indulge.

But when you ask someone about what is in a dish and how they made it, let them know that you'd love to try their dish but you're gluten-intolerant and wanted to ask a couple questions first. It's important they know you're gluten-intolerant because they will be extra careful to disclose all information (and won't be offended that you're asking about their food). Be prepared to explain to them what gluten is because this may be their first time hearing of it.

Caution: Simply asking "Did you use flour in this?" is not sufficient—you'll need to ask the person to name every ingredient in the recipe. This could be a bit awkward depending on the situation, but if you want to eat a mystery dish, you have to be a gluten sleuth. As they recite the ingredients, eliminate what you know to be safe and keep track of the ingredients you need to ask more about. Perhaps the host can show you the bottle or box they used and you can scan the ingredient list. Or if they have the recipe handy they could show it to you. And then don't forget to ask about cross-contact.

How do you navigate around possible cross-contact issues in a dish prepared by someone else?

As more people adopt the gluten-free lifestyle, being inquisitive about foods at social gatherings will become more commonplace. But initially, from the perspective of social graces, it seems a bit awkward to be so nosey about something someone has so generously made for people to enjoy. But you have no choice but to inquire if you want to eat safely at events. With practice, the questions you ask will seem more natural and part of your social-eating routine, and maybe even become the topic of an interesting conversation.

After you've determined that a dish at a party was made with gluten-free ingredients, you can't be 100 percent certain until you ask about cross-contact. This step will depend on your level of gluten-intolerance. You may feel that asking questions about preparation may be too intrusive and uncomfortable in a social situation particularly with someone you don't know. But before making the final decision to partake, think about how the dish was prepared and what equipment and utensils may have been used. Think about the steps you would take to avoid cross-contact in your home and what you would have done if you were making the dish. It's possible the person who made it was not as thorough as you would be—even likely, as they probably aren't used to cooking gluten-free dishes. Ask about how the dish was prepared, eat the dish based on your educated guess that it's safe, or avoid eating the food entirely.

What should you do about the wedding and birthday cake?

If it's your wedding, the good news is you can have your gluten-free cake and eat it too. While it may be difficult finding a bakery in your town that can make a wedding cake using different gluten-free flours, most bakeries will know how to make a chocolate flourless cake or Ganache-style cake. If this style of cake suits your taste, special order it with the first tier being the gluten-free version that you and your spouse can share. You can order the other tiers of the cake for your guests using the bakery's traditional cake recipes.

Or try to find a bakery that has gluten-free cake recipes or who would be willing to accommodate your needs by making a gluten-free cake from a recipe you provide. Offer suggestions on where they can purchase the flours and starches. But expect to pay more for your cake than you otherwise would. Gluten-free flours are more expensive, larger quantities will be used and the price will be passed on to you.

In either case, don't forget to ask your bakery about how they will avoid cross-contact with gluten and meet your standards. Chances are they will not have dedicated space and will need to know something about the protocol. Don't be bashful in sharing steps for them to follow.

And when you're attending a wedding other than your own, arrive with the expectation that you won't be able to partake. The upside? Just think about the calories you will save. Then, of course, this is a delicious excuse to have your own gluten-free cake waiting for you at home after the wedding. Thoughts of digging in after the reception will give you something to look forward to. The same advice applies for attending birthday parties other than your own.

What are suggestions for gluten-free foods and snacks for backpacking and camping trips?

Eating gluten-free in the great outdoors can be one of the most challenging aspects of the lifestyle, if not more challenging than traveling abroad. This will pose some unique challenges to the camping and biking enthusiasts among you. Unfortunately, outdoor recreation stores do not carry a wide variety of foods designed specifically for a gluten-free diet. Nor are there an abundance of companies that supply those nifty vacuum sealed packet meals where you just add water and stir in gluten-free varieties. Until that day comes, and it could be a long wait, you must rely on your creativity and a trip to the grocery store to make your own portable goods.

The list below provides ideas for gluten-free snacks and meals that you can carry in your backpack.

- Nuts such as almonds, Brazil nuts, cashews, and peanuts
- Dried fruits, such as apricots, cranberries, raisins, figs, pineapple rings, apple rings, dates, and mangos
- Gluten-free potato chips, corn chips, crackers, granola, pretzels, cereal, and rice cakes
- Make your own trail mix using your favorite nuts, dried fruits, and gluten-free chocolate chips.
- Small cans (pop tops preferable) of gluten-free meats such a chicken, salmon, and tuna
- Nutrition bars—you can't bring too many of these!
- Fruit in baby cans or plastic containers such as peaches, pineapple, applesauce, or fruit medleys
- Sandwiches using premade gluten-free pancakes, waffles (won't crumble!), or other ingenious, unconventional gluten-free bread slices
- Fruit Leather and gluten-free chocolate bars
- Gluten-free beef or bison jerky
- Prebaked yams or potatoes (if you don't mind eating them cold)
- Consider making your own gluten-free entrees at home, then freeze them in plastic containers—they should be thawed just in time for lunch.
- Make a gluten-free pizza, freeze, and bring the slices.
- Get gluten-free soup mixes in a packet, and use hot water from a thermos to "cook" them.
- My Own Meals, Inc. offers five gluten-free military-style MREs in their special diets category (www.myownmeals.com).

Can you eat gluten-free at the movies, amusement parks, and sporting events?

While going gluten-free doesn't mean entertainment-free, the answer to this question may not be all that entertaining to you. Your chances of finding gluten-free foods at places such as movie theaters, amusement parks, sports arenas, concert halls, park concerts, theatres, shopping malls, video arcades, etc. are extremely slim. Plus, these events are not the best places to read ingredient labels on boxes from the candy case or to ask the cashier to investigate ingredients for you with lines of people behind you.

The majority of foods sold at these venues have gluten. You'll typically find pretzels, hot dogs, hamburgers, corn dogs, ice cream cones, pizza, burritos, and similarly unsuitable foods. But even if a hamburger without the bun is all you can eat, the cross-contact issue prevalent at these venues should be enough to discourage you from making the purchase. Even foods that appear as though they would be gluten-free should raise your eyebrows. Such decoy foods can include corn chips (could have shared oil used to fry gluten-based products), popcorn (could have been seasoned with a butter-flavored seasoning that uses wheat flour as a filler or to prevent clumping), ice cream (could have wheat-based ingredients for thickeners or candy ingredients like cookie chunks), or corn dogs (will have a breading that contains wheat flour, not to mention hidden fillers in the meat). And many candy bars have gluten. Unless you've done your investigative work beforehand and know what's gluten-free, try to eat a good meal prior to going to the event and consider bringing some of your own gluten-free snacks to enjoy.

Should you let your boss and coworkers know about your gluten-intolerance?

It's entirely up to you on how much personal information you like to share with the people you work with, but there are a few things to keep in mind if you choose to keep your gluten-intolerance a secret. If your boss likes to throw surprise parties and buys you a birthday cake with your name drawn on the top in colorful frosting, you'll have to explain why you can't have any. This is obviously a potentially embarrassing situation.

A similar uncomfortable scenario could result when your boss or a coworker brings you a holiday gift of gluten-filled goodies and you won't be able to comment on how delicious the gift was because of course you weren't able to eat them. Or the nice coworker who comes to you and says "I brought you a chocolate chip muffin from the coffee shop downstairs . . ." or the boss who orders a pizza lunch for the group—either way you will have some explaining to do.

Situations such as these will eventually present themselves in the workplace. The best advice is to be open and honest as soon as possible with as many people as you think is necessary, particularly the boss and close staff. This will help you avoid some potentially embarrassing situations in the future. Plus, by sharing the information with them, they may even go out of their way to surprise you with a gluten-free cake for your birthday! It's in your best interest to make sure there are at least a few crucial people at work who know about your intolerance.

How do you avoid cross-contact with gluten at work?

When plates, pans, and silverware are shared in an office, you will not know for certain how well they were cleaned before being made available to use again. Without proper cleaning, it's possible that residual gluten could be left behind in a corner or crevice and if you can't tolerate a trace without getting sick, consider bringing your own things to use or re-cleaning anything you use. This will at least eliminate any suspicion and bring peace of mind.

Be cautious of the usual lunch room suspects such as the community toaster, microwave oven, and cutting board. Workplace lunch rooms are not known for their cleanliness, and you need to be concerned with the potential for cross-contact if you use this equipment. Also, don't forget about the infamous dish towel that everyone uses to dry their dishes. It could have been used to wipe away crumbs on the table from the morning coffee cake.

It's best not to be tempted by foods that are available for anyone in the community refrigerator. While something may appear to be gluten-free, you won't know how it was prepared and what hidden issues it may hold.

At office potlucks, try to be the first in line. This way you can select the foods you can eat and won't run the risk of any cross-contact service issues, like the spoon from the pasta salad accidentally making its way into the fruit salad bowl.

How can you best handle business meetings at restaurants?

If breakfast, lunch or dinner meetings with coworkers or business associates are common practice in your line of work, there will be a variety of scenarios where you'll feel like you're on the spot, rushed, out of your comfort zone, and under the magnifying glass. But again, situations can be best navigated when you have an idea of what to expect and are prepared in advance. Group engagements can often be more uncomfortable than one-on-one meetings.

Scenario #1

You're in an unfamiliar restaurant, it takes you a while to read the menu for gluten-free options, your coworkers are ready to order and get on with the meeting, but you're still trying to make a decision and asking the server questions about the menu. If you haven't let people know about your gluten-intolerance before now, their patience level may not be what it would otherwise be.

Tip: Right after or before everyone sits down, excuse yourself to visit the restroom and conveniently ask the hostess for a menu to take a look at it and get a jump start. Ask if they can recommend gluten-free options. By the time you return to the table, you may have an idea of what you're going to order.

Scenario #2
When you have a meeting at a restaurant scheduled in advance, you have time to call ahead to ask about the menu. Get an idea of what you can order and what to avoid. By the time the engagement rolls around, you can order efficiently and those who accompany you will never know the difference.

   Tip: If your research concludes there will be virtually nothing you can eat at the selected venue, prepare to eat light that day or make a recommendation to switch restaurants.

Scenario #3
Know the restaurants in your business district well and have a list of those you can eat at, as well as those that are not favorable to your diet. When you have to schedule a meeting, you can make recommendations or if someone else is taking the lead, you can guide the situation in your favor.

   Tip: Gather copies of gluten-free menus from nearby restaurants that you like and keep them on file in your office for easy reference when the need to suggest a restaurant arises.

What are some gluten-free snack suggestions for the office?

If you like to keep snacks at your desk, there are many gluten-free delights you can keep at the ready in your drawer. There are two categories of gluten-free snacks: those that can remain in your desk for several days if not weeks, and those you can stock fresh each day. Having a supply of quick-grab, mini-munchies such as gluten-free crackers, cookies, rice cakes, and chocolate will help quell mild snack cravings whenever they arise. However, for the five-alarm snack emergencies, it's best to have fresh, generally refrigerated food at your disposal.

Some ideas to get you thinking outside the cookie jar include:

- Make a gluten-free pizza at home with a fresh hand-made crust and complete with your favorite toppings. After baking, cut it into small snack-size slices and place in baggies for easy transport to the office. Microwave or enjoy cold when the craving strikes.
- Bring containers of spreads like nut butter, jelly, and cream cheese to keep at work to slather on rice cakes, premade pancakes, or dried fruit like apricots and figs. Pancakes or waffles make a great substitute for sliced bread even when cool after being in the refrigerator!
- Create mini-meal snacks that contain a nice combination of carbohydrate and protein, such as cracker sandwiches made with cheese slices and a healthy gluten-free lunch meat or hummus.
- Bring a leftover meal you can spread throughout the day and just scoop out and microwave portions as you need them.

Tip: A protein-carbo combo may be more satisfying in between meals than a protein or carbohydrate will all by itself. Have fresh fruit slices and veggie sticks or freshly made gluten-free trail mix ready to grab out of a baggie.

Chapter 16

HEALTH AND NUTRITION: LOOKING BEYOND GLUTEN FOR BETTER HEALTH

- Is a gluten-free diet healthy?
- Can you discover other food sensitivities on a gluten-free diet?
- Will you lose or gain weight on a gluten-free diet?
- If you feel sick occasionally on a gluten-free diet, what could be the problem?
- Are your bones healthy?
- How can you manage and improve bone density?
- How much calcium do you need?
- Can the introduction of gluten to a baby's diet precipitate celiac disease?
- Is there a link between autism and celiac disease?
- What if you know more about celiac disease and gluten-intolerance than your doctor does?
- How does a positive diagnosis for celiac disease affect your health insurance coverage in the future?
- If you have been denied health insurance because of celiac disease, how can you help reverse the decision?
- How can you live gluten-free in a hospital?
- Are you safe visiting the dentist?
- Will you miss valuable nutrients by eliminating wheat/gluten from your diet?
- What are the most nutritious gluten-free flours?
- What can help improve the nutritional value of gluten-free baked goods?
- Will you feel good on a gluten-free diet?
- What are the signs of a poor gluten-free diet?
- How can you boost your gluten-free diet with fiber?

Is a gluten-free diet healthy?

When looking at the nutritional profiles of the majority of products made by gluten-free product companies, you will notice a theme. There is a widespread commitment to using natural ingredients, many of which are organic. Plus, when you have to avoid many of the highly processed foods that contain gluten, you find that your diet naturally gravitates toward more healthy choices. Consequently, a gluten-free diet is considered a healthy diet because of its tendency to steer you in the direction of healthy foods and when it eliminates the key ingredient you must avoid it's automatically healthier for you!

Naturally, if you buy most of your foods at natural food markets (where the majority of gluten-free products will be found), your choices will be healthier because of what these stores choose *not* to carry. The stores help you make healthy choices. However, as with any diet, there are red flags to watch for and your gluten-free diet can vary on the healthy scale.

Many foods can be designated as gluten-free, but may not have a healthy nutritional profile. If your diet consists largely of processed canned foods and frozen dinners in addition to foods that are high in sugar, refined ingredients, and unhealthy fats despite being gluten-free, your diet can't be considered healthy. Also, watch out for regular use of gluten-free baked products and mixes that contain primarily white ingredients, such as white rice flour, tapioca flour, and potato flour, or if sugar is listed as the first ingredient. If your daily carbohydrate intake consists mostly of nutrient-poor gluten-free ingredients, your diet can suffer. So, while a gluten-free diet is considered to be a healthy diet overall, you are still responsible for making good choices to keep it that way.

Can you discover other food sensitivities on a gluten-free diet?

A gluten-free diet is unique because it introduces you to a broad spectrum of other ingredients, many of which you may never have tried before such as amaranth, buckwheat, millet, quinoa, sorghum, and teff. These are key staples in gluten-free cuisine beyond rice, corn and potatoes, and they are being used more extensively as the gluten-free diet continues to gain prominence and companies develop new gluten-free products. But these ingredients are often new nutritional components to someone embarking upon a gluten-free diet, and it's within the realm of possibility you could be sensitive to one of these new additions.

When cooking and baking the gluten-free way, you naturally become more adventurous and experimental. And with gluten off the radar as a possible culprit, you have a clean slate to clearly determine how other ingredients affect you. For example, flours made from tree nuts are incorporated into gluten-free products and baking. If you have a tree nut allergy you may be sensitive to flour derived from a tree nut. Teff, a tiny nutritious grain native to northern Africa, contains natural yeast and if you're sensitive to yeast, you may have a reaction to teff.

Being on a gluten-free diet naturally makes you more aware of your body and how you react to different foods. Simply monitor how you feel after eating ingredients you have never tried before, make any connections you can, and avoid anything you don't feel is right for you.

Will you lose or gain weight on a gluten-free diet?

The word "diet" is used in a variety of contexts, many of which are driven by the latest of the lose-weight-quick fads. The word is often associated directly, if not subliminally, with losing weight. Diets are popularly known as ways to help you shed those unwanted pounds!

But the word "diet" is also associated with the combinations and nutritional profiles of selected foods you eat over the course of time to promote health, not a crash or short-term program to drop some pounds. While a gluten-free diet is restrictive in one sense (eliminating gluten), it is not a short-term approach but a life-long commitment.

The gluten-free diet is not a fad or a program designed to help you lose weight. Frankly, it's designed to save your life, particularly if you have celiac disease. But asking if you will lose or gain weight on the diet is a valid question. You should consult your doctor or nutritionist on how the diet will apply to your individual situation.

However, a gluten-free diet can promote weight loss in some individuals by virtue of eating less processed foods and enjoying the more natural, wholesome gluten-free foods available. Also, when the body is rejecting gluten, its metabolism can't possibly be at peak performance because it's not properly absorbing nutrients. When your metabolism properly regulates itself, losing weight may be a possible result.

However, gaining weight on a gluten-free diet is possible if you consume too many high-carb, high-sugar, low-fiber foods. As with any diet, poor food choices will not do much for weight management. Losing, gaining or maintaining weight on a gluten-free diet varies from person to person.

If you feel sick occasionally on a gluten-free diet, what could be the problem?

Once you eliminate gluten from your diet, it's expected you will no longer experience the uncomfortable symptoms you once had associated with ingesting gluten. It's commonly reported that people feel like a new person after adopting a gluten-free diet. If you have eliminated gluten from your diet but you still don't feel your best at times, there may be another problem that hasn't been discovered.

Consult your doctor for appropriate guidance, but it could be something as simple as:

- You may be getting traces of gluten somewhere, perhaps through cross-contamination in packaged food products. Double-check your vigilance to the diet.
- It's common to suspect that, when you feel bad after eating a meal at a restaurant, you could have ingested gluten via cross-contamination. While it's possible this may have occurred, you may be reacting to an ingredient you've never tried before that disagrees with you, or it could be a poor food handling issue.
- Some people experience chronic constipation as a symptom of their gluten-intolerance. However, if constipation remains a problem after being gluten-free for a period of time, it could be a sign of not getting enough exercise and fiber in the diet.
- You may be experiencing reactions to other foods you have not yet eliminated from your diet because you haven't realized they're the cause. You may not know about the other food sensitivity because its symptoms were masked or overridden by the symptoms associated with gluten.

Are your bones healthy?

Your bone health is due to your own personal calcium-economics. Envision your skeleton, made up of over three hundred bones, as a bank where the currency is calcium, vitamin D, and minerals essential for bone health. Throughout your life you make savings deposits of calcium through the foods you eat. After your body absorbs the calcium it requires for normal functions, the additional calcium left-over is then used to make a savings deposit into your skeleton. These savings deposits help build and maintain bone density. But after the additional calcium is stored in the skeleton, if there is any excess calcium your skeleton does not need it will be eliminated through the urine as a payout with no physical benefit, similar to throwing money down the drain. This is why monitoring calcium supplement dosage and timing is important: Taking too much calcium in one dose will produce excess that will be wasted through excretion.

Naturally, calcium savings deposits are closely related to the diet. If the diet is sufficient in calcium, the savings deposits should be at a healthy amount. However, the body's ability to absorb calcium is inherently linked to the digestive system. When the digestive system does not work properly, as in the case of celiac disease, complications with calcium absorption can occur and impact the body's calcium-economics. In fact, malabsorption issues relating to celiac disease can place the body into a perpetual calcium savings withdrawal mode, where it takes out a loan on your account to serve the needs of the rest of the body. This calcium deficit can occur regardless of age when the disease is left unchecked and a strict gluten-free diet is not being followed. Research suggests there is a clear link between celiac disease and poor bone density, which can result in conditions such as osteoporosis, osteopenia, or decalcified bones known as osteomalacia.

Bone density problems are a prevalent debilitating effect of untreated celiac disease. If you have been diagnosed with celiac disease or if you highly suspect you have the disease and have not been tested, consult with your doctor on taking a panel of blood tests that reveal how well your blood holds onto the calcium it needs and/or a bone mineral density test. This test will reveal the health and density of your bones in comparison to standards of normal bone density for your age. The results will determine the next step.

How can you manage and improve bone density?

Whether you have celiac disease or not, bone health should be on your radar. Up through young adult life, the body's skeleton develops based on your calcium savings rate over the years. But then it plateaus and you are responsible for maintaining what you've built by continuing to save without making any withdrawals. If you have celiac disease and your bone health is not where it should be, you can take action to help manage the condition and start building bone mass. In some cases, doctors will prescribe drugs to help improve bone density. But the good news is that much of your bone health can be within your control!

You can boost your calcium level with a gluten-free diet. If you have celiac disease, going on a balanced gluten-free diet will heal the villi in your small intestine and should correct any malabsorption issues you had, thus making proper absorption of calcium, vitamin D, and magnesium possible.

Then, of course, you have to make the calcium deposits. Even when you're on a gluten-free diet, if you don't give the body the calcium it needs daily, there will be no savings made. Focus on sources rich in calcium, including foods such as green leafy vegetables, nuts, salmon with edible bones, and even dairy products if they're right for you. When you're reading labels for gluten, read for calcium too!

It can be challenging to consume your daily calcium and vitamin D requirements through foods alone, so gluten-free nutritional calcium supplements can help close the gap and get you where you need to be daily. And the sun is a wonderful source of vitamin D. If you live in a region and climate that allows you to receive several minutes of sunscreen-protected sunshine a day, take advantage and enjoy.

Last but not least, exercise! Exercising builds bones. If you regularly exercise, congratulations and keep up the good work. If you don't, incorporate some form of weight bearing exercise into your routine. Consult with your doctor on an exercise regimen that's best for you before you start.

How much calcium do you need?

According to Dr. Peter Green in his book *Celiac Disease, A Hidden Epidemic*, females in their early fifties should take 1,000 to 1,200 milligrams of calcium a day and males should take 800 to 1,200 milligrams of calcium a day. Younger, premenopausal women should take 1,000 milligrams of calcium a day. Dr. Green also recommends a ladder of vitamin D based on age. Women before menopause should take 200 International Units (IU) a day, women during menopause should up the amount to 400 IU a day, and women after menopause should increase to 600 IU a day. On the other hand, men, regardless of age, should take 400 IU a day.

Tip: Remember, vitamin D is important for proper absorption of calcium. Spread your calcium intake appropriately throughout the day. Your body can absorb no more than 500 to 600 milligrams in one dose, and it needs vitamin D to do it.

Can the introduction of gluten to a baby's diet precipitate celiac disease?

More attention is now being given to the timing of introducing wheat and gluten-based foods to babies, and how that timing may impact whether or not babies genetically predisposed to celiac disease will develop the disease. If gluten is introduced too early or too late, the child's risk of developing the disease may increase.

It's clear at this point that the research is only suggestive and much remains to be studied. But initial research findings indicate that babies introduced to gluten within their first three months were at higher risk of developing the disease than babies who were first introduced to gluten between four to six months of age. And babies who are first introduced to gluten after seven months have a marginally increased rate of developing the disease. These findings suggest an optimal window of time for introducing gluten to the diet—between four and six months of age. Research also suggests that breast feeding in conjunction with introducing gluten may have an effect on preventing the development of celiac disease in genetically predisposed babies. Regardless of the research, consult your doctor on the best way to introduce gluten into your baby's diet.

Is there a link between autism and celiac disease?

Putting children with autism on the gluten-free/casein-free diet is an intervention measure which has been found to have positive effects on autistic behavioral problems. It's common that children with autism have various food sensitivities and gastrointestinal symptoms, particularly in relation to grains. However, recent research supported by Tehran University of Medical Sciences suggests there is no link between autism and celiac disease. Of the thirty-four children studied, it was found they were at no more risk for developing celiac disease than children who do not have autism. While a gluten-free diet is found to be beneficial for those with autism in managing behavioral symptoms, no direct link to gluten-intolerance is suggested. This research counters the previously considered links between the two conditions.

What if you know more about celiac disease and gluten-intolerance than your doctor does?

It's a rare case when you find yourself more knowledgeable about a medical subject than your doctor. But as awareness of celiac disease and gluten-intolerance continues to increase among the general population, this phenomenon is on the rise. When individuals suspect they've figured out the cause of their condition, they can be insatiable for information. After reading books and newsletters on the topic, consuming prolific amounts of information via the Internet, and participating in blogs, patient-consumers are becoming information savvy. As a result, it's becoming more common for patients to have more information than their own doctor on gluten-intolerance, and they may be able to provide facts the doctor doesn't know. The medical community is becoming more and more uniform in their knowledge of the condition, but until there is wide-spread expertise on the matter, it won't hurt to do some independent research.

If you find yourself more knowledgeable on celiac disease or gluten-intolerance than your doctor, consider it a blessing in disguise and choose from these two primary options:

Option #1
If you feel that your doctor is not as knowledgeable as you are about celiac disease, gluten-intolerance, and food sensitivities in general, this is a good sign to find another doctor. This can open the door for you to be referred to an excellent gastroenterologist. The reality is that you can't expect your general physician to know all conditions equally, and there are times when a specialist is needed.

Option #2
If you like your current doctor and they are somewhat knowledge-able about the condition, your research can help create a good synergy with your doctor and enable you to double-check informa-tion. For example: Let's say you've read somewhere reliable that, in order for blood work to be accurate, it's imperative that you consume gluten for a period of time before the test. But if you've been gluten-free for more than six months now and your doctor orders the tests without asking you to take the "gluten challenge" (Chapter One) you have grounds to ask why not and to let them know what you know.

How does a positive diagnosis for celiac disease affect your health insurance coverage in the future?

The "pre-existing condition" is a pivotal decision-making factor for insurance companies when granting or denying health insurance coverage to an individual. People have been denied health insurance countless times because of a "pre-existing condition," including celiac disease, and many times the insurance company does not want to assume the possible health care costs associated with the individual who has the condition. Without getting into the reasons why you can be denied coverage, many of which can be infuriating, the answer is yes: you could be denied health insurance coverage in the future as a result of being diagnosed with celiac disease.

If you are currently covered by health insurance and have just been diagnosed, your coverage will remain with full benefits. The concern arises when you decide to apply for insurance coverage on your own, without the umbrella of assistance that comes with a workplace-sponsored insurance program. If you suspect you have celiac disease and would like to get tested, you need to ask yourself: Would a positive diagnosis be worth the risk of possibly being denied insurance coverage later in life? If you've been living a gluten-free diet and feel remarkably better than you ever have and have no intentions of going back, but don't have a positive medical diagnosis, you have to decide if you want the diagnosis on your medical record.

Wanting to know if you have celiac disease or if your children have it is natural. But unfortunately, the way the insurance structure is, getting diagnosed and getting that "pre-existing condition" mark is a personal decision only you can make. Just knowing a gluten-free diet works well for you or your children may be all you need to know, and a positive medical diagnosis is not worth the possible future frustrations when filing for a private health insurance coverage.

If you have been denied health insurance because of celiac disease, how can you help reverse the decision?

If you have been denied health insurance coverage because of celiac disease, chances are it was by a smaller insurance company that carries higher liability because of less members paying into the till and a higher risk rate of health claims. Without getting into the discussion about whether it's fair or not to deny someone with a "pre-existing condition," let it suffice to say that you are encouraged to put your best effort forward to state that your case *should* be accepted.

Even though being diagnosed with celiac disease becomes a "pre-existing condition" in the eyes of an insurance company, it's a diagnosis with the silver lining of preventative maintenance. Left undiagnosed and not managed through a permanent gluten-free diet, celiac disease can lead to further and more serious complications, thus claims, which you now have a greater chance of avoiding. Any insurance company should look at a celiac diagnosis, particularly early diagnosis without the presence of long-term complications, as a prognosis for better health, not the other way around.

A gluten-free diet can be considered one of the healthiest diets around, and it's quite possible that other nonceliac conditions may be avoided or better managed—a gluten-free diet has been found to help other conditions such as arthritis, multiple sclerosis, autism, and diabetes. Your diagnosis and subsequent diet could possibly reduce the risk of future claims. And if an insurance company says they can't be sure you're complying with the diet as grounds for denial, offer to periodically undergo testing for antibodies and the results will reveal your compliance!

Don't delay. Call your insurance company to ask for the contact information of the appropriate person to send a letter to, state your case adamantly, and have your situation rereviewed and reconsidered.

How can you live gluten-free in a hospital?

It's ironic that eating gluten-free in a hospital can be a challenge, but just as with restaurants, gluten-free diet awareness and procedures vary. When you're a patient, you will need to be prepared to educate your care team about your gluten-free diet needs. This includes your doctor, nurse, dietician, and cafeteria manager.

When being admitted to a hospital, you will be asked about your allergies. Even though celiac disease or gluten-intolerance is not an "allergy" to gluten, hospital staffs understand what the term allergy means and it's important to include gluten in the allergy category for your medical chart. You may want to clarify "gluten" by also saying wheat, barely, rye, and oats (oats in a hospital will most likely be contaminated, so mention them!).

Make a card for your wallet that includes a list of your allergies and intolerances, including gluten. Bring a document that explains celiac disease and the foods you can't eat. This can be given to members of your care team to include in your chart for quick reference, as well as passed to the cafeteria personnel responsible for preparing your meals. Also, make sure that the person responsible for submitting your prescriptions asks the pharmacist to check for gluten in each medication.

If you have time on your side before being admitted to a hospital (if you're having a baby, a scheduled surgery, or any other preplanned hospital stay), call ahead to speak with the appropriate person who can help facilitate gluten-free meals for you in advance.

But always take some gluten-free foods with you, including snacks you can keep in your room and foods that can be prepared for you, like creamy rice cereal or even pure, gluten-free oatmeal if you can tolerate the oats.

On the other hand, if you are visiting someone in the hospital and need to eat there, approach the situation as you would with cafeterias, bars, restaurants, and salad bars—extremely proactive and cautious.

Are you safe visiting the dentist?

Living gluten-free doesn't stop with avoiding foods with gluten. It's also important to be mindful of dental hygiene products when you visit the dentist. While most dental products are gluten-free, some may not be, so you need to double-check with your dentist. To be safe, call your dentist several days before your next visit to let them know you are gluten-intolerant and you would like them to research the gluten-free status of the products they will be using on you. They may be unfamiliar with gluten and could call the product manufacturers to confirm, which could take some time.

Aside from the products used in cleaning and other procedures, be watchful of gloves. Although most would be coated in corn starch, some latex or vinyl gloves may be coated with oat flour and it will not be pure oat flour, but contaminated oat flour. Ask your dentist to use non-powdered gloves to be safe.

Will you miss valuable nutrients by eliminating wheat/gluten from your diet?

While wheat, barley, rye, and cross-contaminated oats are considered dangerous grains to those who can't digest them properly, they are by nature filled with valuable nutrition. For example, whole wheat in its whole grain state or when stone ground into flour is naturally packed with protein and fiber. When you eliminate whole wheat from your lifestyle, you automatically eliminate its nutrients and will need to find gluten-free replacements with similar nutritional features.

But when transitioning to a gluten-free diet, it's easy to get in trouble from the start, feasting upon highly-refined, high-carbohydrate gluten-free foods made from white rice flour, potato flour, tapioca starch, and lots of sugar. Even though these flours work well functionally within gluten-free baked goods and products, they alone are not equivalent replacements for the nutrition whole wheat flour provides.

So, what are you missing? Whole wheat flour has 16 grams of protein per cup, while white rice flour has 8 grams per cup and tapioca flour has zero grams per cup. Wheat flour has 12 grams of dietary fiber, whereas white rice flour has 4 grams of dietary fiber per cup and tapioca flour has zero grams. By comparing these figures, it's clear that a gluten-free diet is susceptible to a nutritional deficiency if other whole grains and flours are not incorporated.

Try to include higher protein, higher fiber gluten-free grains and flours in your diet.

Quinoa, amaranth, teff, and millet are sound replacements for wheat, barley, and rye. Even pure, gluten-free oats are an option if you have determined you can tolerate oats. Also, flours made from these grains will have a higher nutritional value when used in baked goods. Sorghum flour is also known for its wheat-like properties in baking and has a high nutritional value similar to wheat.

What are the most nutritious gluten-free flours?

Figures vary from manufacturer to manufacturer, but in general, whole wheat flour is high in protein and fiber, packing 16 grams of protein and 15 grams of fiber per one cup of flour. Refined white flour has 16 grams of protein, but the fiber drops to only 4 grams. Protein is not only a vital nutrient for the diet, it's also elemental for successful baking—it's what keeps the stuff from crumbling apart.

When eliminating the wheat flour from your diet, it's easy to proportionally decrease your protein and fiber intake unless it's replaced with other nutritious gluten-free flours. There are a number of gluten-free flours that rank higher in protein and fiber than wheat flour.

Flours made from nuts and beans are highly nutritious. For example, one cup of almond flour has 23.6 grams of protein and 14.7 grams of fiber. Bean flours (Chickpea, Garfava, Navy, Pinto, and White) range between 23.2 to 34.9 grams of protein and 12 to 32 grams of fiber. Amaranth flour has a 19.5 and 12.6 protein/fiber ratio. Soy flour with no fat removed tops the chart at 47 grams of protein and 17.5 grams of fiber. Montina, also known as Indian Ricegrass, ranks high with 25.5 grams of protein and 36 grams of fiber. Sorghum flour is considered to be highly nutritious flour and comes closest to replicating the baking attributes of wheat flour, with 16 grams of protein per one cup.

Also, did you know flours have calcium? Values vary from flour to flour, but for comparison purposes, wheat flour has 41 mg of calcium per one cup flour, while almond flour has 289 mg, teff flour has 239 mg, amaranth comes in at 207 mg, soy comes in at 173 mg and flax meal has 332 mg.

Resources: Shelley Case, *The Gluten-Free Diet*, individual manufacturers.

What can help improve the nutritional value of gluten-free baked goods?

When making your own gluten-free baked goods at home or looking at ingredient labels on packaged products in the store, the following list can provide some directional check points for boosting nutritional value. Consult gluten-free cookbooks for advice on appropriate ratios to yield the additional nutritional value you want without compromising on the baking performance.

- Flours higher in protein and fiber such as amaranth, quinoa, teff, sorghum, navy bean, pinto bean, and nut flours
- Less reliance on white flours and starches
- By-products of rice flour production such as rice polish and rice bran.

- Brown rice is more nutritious than white rice.
- Natural, unrefined sweeteners and fruit pastes, or purees are a better choice than refined white sugar.
- For lower fat content, substitute some applesauce or fruit puree for oil.
- Add fruit such as raisins, cranberries, cherries, and blueberries.
- Add flax seeds or flaxseed meal in small quantities.
- Use high quality, nutritious vegetable oils in lieu of butter.
- Add fruit juice concentrates.
- Incorporate flakes of amaranth or quinoa.
- For sugar-free baking, consider Xylotol, a natural sweetener made from birch trees.

Will you feel good on a gluten-free diet?

Naturally, feeling good is a relative term. However, there are a variety of scenarios that can result from adopting a gluten-free diet. Keep in mind that the time it takes to feel better on the diet is also relative to the individual.

If you have celiac disease or gluten-intolerance and experience severe or chronic physical reactions to gluten, you will probably feel almost immediately better on a gluten-free diet. Once the culprit is removed, your body can breathe a sigh of relief and restore its way to a healthier you. Many people feel like they have been given a new lease on life when they begin a gluten-free diet.

If you have dermatitis herpetiformis and experience severe skin irritations as a result of ingesting gluten, you will feel better on a gluten-free diet after the skin is healed. Feeling good may take longer for the individual with this condition if current skin lesions have to heal, but this is often aided by medication. Dapsone is the primary medication used to treat dermatitis herpetiformis and must be prescribed by a doctor.

If you do not feel severe or chronic physical symptoms as a result of ingesting gluten but are diagnosed with celiac disease, the damage is "silent" and you may not experience a dramatic, newfound sense of well-being on a gluten-free diet. In fact, you may find sticking to the diet to be a tough and cruel measure. People for whom gluten does not produce a severe reaction may have a much harder time sticking to the lifestyle, as they do not have immediate repercussions from breaking it.

If you strictly follow a gluten-free diet, but have other food intolerances that happen to be gluten-free of which you are unaware, it's possible you won't feel good on such a diet.

If you follow a gluten-free diet and your symptoms have dissipated, but you do not have a healthy diet and lack proper exercise, you may not feel good on a gluten-free diet despite the fact that it's working in your favor to fight the disease.

If you are not gluten-intolerant or gluten-sensitive but choose to follow a gluten-free diet, chances are you will feel great, because this is generally a healthy diet, perhaps healthier than what you were used to.

What are the signs of a poor gluten-free diet?

It's common to think that a gluten-free diet is automatically a healthy diet. But while it does have its share of nutritional benefits, it can be subject to poor nutrition if not monitored closely. It's easy that in your excitement to find gluten-free foods that you can enjoy you miss out on checking for the valuable nutrients in them.

Contrary to popular belief, you can easily adopt a gluten-free junk-food lifestyle if the majority of foods you eat are high in refined sugar and hydrogenated fats and lacking favorable portions of dietary fiber. Regularity is generally a good indicator of digestive health, and poor regularity on a gluten-free diet can be a sign of not getting enough water, fiber, or exercise.

Some other ways of not getting enough nutrition on a gluten-free diet include: too much reliance on starchy foods such as potatoes, pastas, and breads without a healthy balance of gluten-free whole grains, not eating enough fresh fruits and vegetables, eating most of your foods from a can or a package and not enough raw foods, or too many foods with just white flours or too much sugar. As with any other diet, you need to make sure your nutritional bases are covered.

How can you boost your gluten-free diet with fiber?

While it's easy to tell you to eat more fruits and vegetables every day to increase fiber, a gluten-free diet requires a bit more creativity and resourcefulness. You can also add fiber to your diet by cutting back or subtracting low-fiber foods such as highly refined baked goods made from low-fiber flours. Other fiber-boosting suggestions include:

- Establish a daily menu plan where at least one meal of the day has a generous portion of a high-fiber gluten-free grain such as brown rice, wild rice, quinoa, amaranth, or teff.
- If your palate welcomes the taste, consider making legumes a staple in your diet. The abundance and versatility of this high-fiber food gives you many meal options to explore.
- Whole grains and legumes can go nicely together in many main dishes or can be complementary side dishes to a meat portion. Plus, you benefit from the protein boost from beans. Beans and rice is a popular pair for making a complete protein.
- Could you replace whole grain brown rice for pasta or potatoes in a traditional recipe? Or look for high-fiber flours to replace low-fiber flours in baked products.
- Try to find ways to add high-fiber flours or seeds to your recipes. Add a small portion of flaxseed meal or rice bran to your flour

blend for a baked good or a skillet delight such as pancakes, sprinkle flaxseeds or sesame seeds over hot cereal. Toasted pumpkin seeds make a high-fiber snack.

- Dried fruits such as figs can be great grazing snacks throughout the day. Dip in nut butter for added protein.
- Find gluten-free crackers that utilize high-fiber flours, grains, and seeds to snack on in between meals.

Chapter 17

PSYCHOLOGY: DEVELOPING COPING STRATEGIES AND MANAGING CRAVINGS

- When beginning a gluten-free diet, what will boost your confidence?
- How can you avoid getting discouraged when starting the gluten-free diet?
- Is it hard to give up the gluten-baked goods?
- Will you always crave the gluten-based foods?
- How do you move through the initial anger stage to acceptance?
- How do you deal with the initial fear of dining out?
- When you get tired of asking questions, what can you do?
- What are good snacks to eat when cravings for gluten hit?
- What are strategies for defeating cravings for gluten-baked foods?
- Will you feel satisfied eating gluten-free?

When beginning a gluten-free diet, what will boost your confidence?

Taking on a gluten-free diet is a life-changing event. Building confidence and making the lifestyle possible for the long haul involves knowing:

- For so many everyday foods you used to eat, you will be able to find a gluten-free version. From breads, pastas, and cereals to cookies, baking mixes, and individual flours, substitution options are available.
- You can find gluten-free products without searching high and low. And with online shopping, ordering gluten-free is just a click away even if you live in a small town.
- The gluten-free food movement is continuing to grow by leaps and bounds. New, delicious, and nutritious products are hitting the shelves regularly. As more companies catch the wave, they will be working hard to produce great tasting products that you can enjoy and trust.
- You can visit many bookstores to find gluten-free cookbooks that will help you cook and bake at home. Or simply type "Gluten-Free Recipes" into your favorite online search engine for an abundance of options.
- Every time you say "no" to gluten, the easier it gets to say no the next time.
- Food labeling rules are being developed that will help you better navigate the grocery store—finding "GF" and "Gluten-Free" on packages will continue to become more common.
- Now you know you don't have to feel ill anymore. Other foods you may have suspected to be the culprit before can now be eaten with confidence.

- More and more restaurants are stepping up to the plate and offering gluten-free options and full menus.
- You can join a local celiac support group and avail yourself of the many resources and educational products they offer.
- You are now a part of a growing community of individuals who are taking the same journey you are. You're not alone!

How can you avoid getting discouraged when starting the gluten-free diet?

Everyone who has adopted the gluten-free diet has been discouraged at some point or another, because the lifestyle does eliminate a bounty of options that was easy to take for granted before going gluten-free. At first it can seem as if you're giving up everything! But as you leave one bounty behind, you make room for another bounty of ingredients, food products, and recipes in your life. And simply recognizing how much better you feel without eating gluten can often be enough to give you all the willpower you need.

Yet, the options around you are not always immediately apparent when you begin this lifetime adventure. The beginning is marked by exploration and experimentation. But the number one key to preventing discouragement is *building and maintaining realistic expectations*. Simply knowing what to expect and understanding the realities of what you will face daily can help you be prepared and to cope. Realistic expectations help keep you on track by knowing what you're options are in any given place, and encouraging you to become proactive in your self-interest.

For example, when you're hungry on a road trip, you can't expect to find a wide variety of gluten-free snacks at gas stations, convenient stores, or airports, so you bring your own. You can't expect to eat gluten-free at a party potluck, so you bring your own food to share. You can't expect your airline flight to serve a gluten-free meal, so you order one in advance.

As you embark upon a gluten-free diet, think about one handy equation for preventing discouragement: For every realistic circumstance you learn and prepare for, you lose a reason to be discouraged and gain an opportunity to become stronger in living the gluten-free life.

Is it hard to give up the gluten-baked goods?

No sugar coated answer is available—at first, it can be a definite challenge to give up gluten-baked goods. Even though your body can't tolerate gluten, cutting it out cold turkey requires an adjustment period. It can be challenging both physically and mentally because many wheat/gluten-based foods are comforting, delicious, and satisfying (even though they made you feel sick). But take heart—it gets easier with time.

When you begin the elimination phase, it's important to remember that you're letting go of the gluten, *not* the foods. You can still have chocolate chip cookies hot from the oven, fluffy pancakes and waffles, piping hot pasta, fresh baked breads, pizza, and more. The only thing missing is the gluten, replaced with other gluten-free flours, grains, and other ingredients.

You will feel so much better living a life without the symptoms provoked by gluten, this feeling will more than compensate for the initial difficulty in giving it up.

Will you always crave the gluten-based foods?

By definition, a craving is a desire or longing for something, and craving the foods you used to eat is a natural part of the process of going gluten-free. In the first few weeks of the diet, your body begins calming down, no longer reacting violently to the gluten, paving the way for further restoration and healing. But you may be fighting the cravings.

Over the years of eating gluten-based foods, particularly your favorite baked goods, your palate became programmed to the taste of wheat in its many varieties. It's no secret that wheat-based baked goods, whether physically in front of you or lingering in your thoughts, have the power to seduce the tummy and palate even when you're not hungry. When beginning a gluten-free diet, the memory of the wheat foods you know and love will still be etched in your palate's memory.

You'll find that many gluten-free products taste different and have a different texture from what you're used to. But you will find gluten-free foods that taste and feel good to you, and with time, your taste buds and olfactory system will adapt and your appreciation of the flavors and textures of gluten-free products will replace your craving for wheat. Then guess what? You may find yourself dealing with cravings for your favorite gluten-free foods!

How do you move through the initial anger stage to acceptance?

Being told by a doctor that you have to follow a gluten-free diet for the rest of your life is not necessarily the type of news that results in joy. In fact, it's quite a natural response to be angry. You may ask "Why me?" or even blame your family tree for the harsh hand with which you've been dealt. Thoughts of what you can no longer eat may seem all pervasive in the beginning, and the hungry, craving stomach rules the mind and emotions. But as healing quickly begins and continues, the mind begins to take control and the stomach eventually follows.

From the beginning, make the choice not to become angry and be determined to be satisfied. Your relationship with food is going to change forever and you have two choices: You can let the restrictive nature of the diet control your life, or you can become proactive and find the abundance and fun in gluten-free living. You get what you focus on.

Approach #1
From the start, actively replace gluten-based foods you used to enjoy with gluten-free versions where possible. The sooner you start experimenting with and enjoying the options available to you, the sooner you'll learn to accept and enjoy them.

Approach #2
Being thankful that you found out now rather than later can move you to the acceptance stage quicker. Feeling better without gluten is a reward that gives you the opportunity to broaden your eating experiences, one you may not have taken otherwise.

Approach #3
Things could be worse. The cure for celiac disease or gluten-intolerance, despite its life changing course, is not about giving up food! You're simply eating different foods, many of which will be new and wonderfully pleasing to you.

Approach #4
A gluten-free diet is considered one of the healthiest diets around. This is an opportunity to make nutritional improvements in your life beyond removing the gluten.

Approach #5
If you like to bake, this is an opportunity to broaden your skills and have fun in adopting new approaches to the art of baking.

How do you deal with the initial fear of dining out?

Once you begin to reap the physical rewards of living gluten-free on the home front, the dining scene may beckon. The last thing you want is to temporarily erase your hard work in avoiding gluten with an unsafe, mistake-prone experience at a restaurant that leaves you feeling ill. Chapter Nine covers the dining scene in detail, but in the beginning, being fearful of dining out is a natural response. But always remember, you are in the driver's seat and it begins with fore-thought and double-checking the service staff's knowledge.

Dining out gets easier the more you do it, but keeping the following tips in mind can lessen your fear of eating in restaurants.

- Call restaurants ahead to inquire about gluten-free menus. These are obviously safer places to start and can be a good way to ease back into the dining scene.
- Even if a restaurant does not have a gluten-free menu, if they are aware of the diet and are happy to accommodate your needs, this can put your mind at ease. Restaurant staffs who are genuinely interested in going the extra mile to render good service can lessen your fear.
- Despite finding a good level of awareness at a restaurant, it never hurts to double-check or test their knowledge against your own. The answers the staff provides you will either boost your confidence or rattle it. Dine at the restaurants that boost your confidence! Leave those that rattle it.
- Do your homework and avoid dining establishments that you know can be a cause for fear either because of the menu or possibilities of cross-contamination in what they serve.

When you get tired of asking questions, what can you do?

If you could save one dollar for every question you'll ask when living gluten-free, you could conceivably enjoy an early retirement. You will get tired of asking questions—it's inevitable. Living gluten-free entails regularly questioning friends, family and restaurant staff, but as you become more accustomed to the diet, there will be more and more things you will be able to figure out on your own.

In the first stage of the diet when you're still learning the ropes, the questions are naturally more frequent. However, with time and trial you'll learn when you can get away without asking a question because your deductive reasoning will have sharpened. However, you will probably always have questions in some situations, and when your enthusiasm or initiative in asking the necessary questions begins to wane or takes a break, your potential for risk increases. Nearly every seasoned gluten-free person can attest to at least one occasion when they didn't ask a question, made an assumption, and got sick as a result. Just one scenario like this will bring about a question-asking renaissance in your life.

But when this red flag appears, it's time to take notice and implement preventative actions. Either fight through your aversion to questioning, or ask others to help you for awhile. For example, your spouse can take over the drill when the server arrives at the table or can call the restaurant ahead of time. Or perhaps it's time to purchase the latest gluten-free product listing from your local support group or national organization to have handy for reference, often relieving you of the responsibility of calling the manufacturer to confirm. Even though you will occasionally get sick of the lifestyle, you have to take the proper steps to protect yourself.

What are good snacks to eat when gluten cravings hit?

If you thought gluten-free meal planning can be challenging at times, finding good gluten-free snacks can be even more so. Snacks are often essential treats in getting through to the next meal period particularly when the cravings strike. Of course, it's easy to suggest healthy snacks such as apple slices or carrots and celery sticks. But let's face reality. Boring!

You might seek solace in eating gluten-free cookies straight from the box, and while they are super for the transition time in adjusting to a life without wheat, over time, you'll be looking for something else more nutritious and substantial. To make great gluten-free snacks, you need a little creativity and forethought. Consider some of the following suggestions that can be made ahead and conveniently packaged in baggies for easy transport. While there are hundreds of other ideas, these may stir your creative juices in the right direction.

- Cracker Sandwiches: Take two gluten-free crackers and create your own fillings. Choose from a variety of ingredients such as gluten-free cream cheese and turkey bacon, almond or peanut butter with preserves, hummus and sliced cucumbers, or egg or crab (not imitation) salad. They are a nice combination of carbohydrate and protein.
- Pancake or Waffle Sandwiches: Make a batch of pancakes or waffles from your favorite gluten-free pancake mix (there are several varieties in the market). Take one or two pancakes or waffles and use them like you would slices of bread combined with your favorite fillings.
- Fruit Muffins: Find a versatile gluten-free baking mix that can make pancakes, muffins, and cookies. Use the muffin recipe and

adjust to add chocolate chips or fruit such as pineapple tidbits, cranberries, or diced peaches.

What are strategies for defeating cravings for gluten-baked foods?

Nobody who has gone gluten-free will ever say the beginning was easy. Cravings are often more an emotional issue, a longing for what you can no longer have, and not an authentic physical hunger. Plus, the memory of the smell and taste of wheat-based baked goods are alive and well in the beginning. You'll want to indulge and take comfort in gluten-free equivalents of your favorite wheat-based goods. Sure it's great to eat fresh fruits and vegetables when cravings strike, but the reality is it's the doughy-sweet goods that will defeat your cravings and satisfy your soul in difficult times.

Think about the times you had cravings for wheat foods before going gluten-free and find your patterns. If you enjoyed cookies in the afternoon at the office, enjoy gluten-free cookies at that time as a replacement. Make a list of the wheat-baked goods you used to eat and find replacements.

Take gluten-free snacks with you wherever you go to help defeat cravings and hunger pangs at the times when they used to pop-up before going gluten-free. Cookies, muffins, brownies, or nutrition/breakfast bars work particularly well when you're on the road traveling, driving to work, shopping, running errands, or after exercising. Don't think of it as adopting an unhealthy routine. This is simply a method to help get you through the initial phase.

Avoid places like bakeries or the grocery aisles that will stir your cravings. When you go to a restaurant, bring a slice of your own gluten-free bread in a baggie to eat with butter at the table, discretely of course. If anyone complains, let them know they should offer a gluten-free option for those who can't eat traditional wheat bread!

As time goes on and your memory for the taste of wheat delights fade (and they will!), you will rely less on this strategy, but in the beginning always have something available that you like.

Will you feel satisfied eating gluten-free?

In the realm of food, "satisfied" can vary with each individual, but you should feel full, nourished, and content after eating. And despite its many challenges, the longer you live gluten-free the more satisfied you become.

Your personal definition of being satisfied will take on new meaning. Your body will no longer grapple with fighting gluten. You will enjoy the foods you eat without feeling uncomfortable symptoms afterward. This in itself is a form of satisfaction that's priceless.

But realistically speaking, when first taking on the challenge of living gluten-free, it's common to feel deprived as well as overwhelmed. In many ways it's like learning a new language or skill. Everywhere you turn, you notice gluten and it reminds you of what you can't have. But living gluten-free opens many doors of satisfaction for you even though you may not recognize them at first. With so many delicious gluten-free versions available of the foods you used to eat, you won't go hungry. Plus, there are different ingredients you will be introduced to. Have you tried teff, amaranth, and quinoa yet? Options abound! You won't like all gluten-free foods, but that's fine. You didn't like all gluten-based foods either.

But remember, if your diet is not balanced and lacks a sound nutritious foundation, you won't feel ultimately satisfied no matter what you eat. Authentic, long-lasting satisfaction comes by eating that which is nourishing to your body. You can design a delicious, nutritious, and satisfying gluten-free lifestyle with thought, planning, and good choices. Simply continue on the adventure to find and eat the foods that satisfy you in healthy ways while not begrudging yourself a little indulgence once in a while.

Conclusion

BRAVE NEW GLUTEN-FREE WORLD: HOPEFUL MUSINGS FOR THE FUTURE

The following list is not factual—at least, not yet. But in the spirit of growth, continual improvement, and promise for an even better gluten-free lifestyle than what is available to us today, these are my predictions/hopes for the future for all of us who continue to live the gluten-free lifestyle and for those who are yet to discover and adopt this incredible way of life. When we look toward the future from the perspective of abundance, options, and optimal health, we create a positive energy today that can make hopes and dreams a reality tomorrow. May this gluten-free manifesto of sorts, written in the future tense, strike a chord within you too as visualizing the possibilities strikes a chord in me everyday. Since living the gluten-free lifestyle for the past seven years, I can glowingly attest that the lifestyle just gets easier and more deliciously abundant every year! And it's wonderful to ponder what is yet to come.

Foods:

More and more emerging small business entrepreneurs continue to develop gluten-free products to serve the growing demand, thus yielding an even wider variety of choices for the gluten-free consumer.

Grocery Shopping:

It's common to find a variety of small food stores in most metropolitan cities which are devoted to carrying an extensive line of gluten-free foods. And larger grocery stores in metropolitan areas have continued to outgrow the small areas of shelf space earlier devoted to gluten-free products and have designated larger sections of floor and shelf space to selling them now. This demand will help make shopping faster and more efficient for those living the gluten-free way of life in the years to come.

Prices:

Prices have decreased for many consumer gluten-free products such as flours and baked goods because the increased demand and volume of gluten-free food product production has allowed manufacturers to decrease the price of the gluten-free ingredients used to make their products. As a result companies and stores can pass their price savings to the consumer, and this will continue to happen as competition in the market thrives.

Food labeling:

Labeling regulations have become more uniform and widespread. The gluten-free consumer can pick up nearly any processed product, glance at the label, and see whether the product is designated as gluten-free without needing to scour the ingredient list or call the food manufacturer to confirm gluten-free status. More companies will be confident in voluntarily labeling their products as gluten-free because they have made the necessary adjustments in their facilities to allow them to claim the designation and not miss out on the gluten-free market demand. More deli counters and food buffets will be easier to navigate with ingredient listings noting any possible allergens in the food and more gluten-free selections will be available overall.

Cookbooks and Television:

A comprehensive selection of gluten-free cookbooks in a variety of cuisines are available in mainstream and independent bookstores. Mainstream television networks broadcast food and lifestyle programs that regularly feature gluten-free cooking and baking segments or full-length features and shows.

Restaurants:

It's commonplace for most restaurants to offer a gluten-free menu, easily make special diet accommodations where necessary, and easily prepare gluten-free meals free of cross-contact. Gluten-free dining is now a cinch.

Culinary Schools:

More culinary schools have incorporated gluten-free baking and cooking courses into their standard curriculum and are now required components for a culinary degree. Chefs have been thoroughly trained and even a Certified Master Gluten-Free Baker program for chefs who want the title has been started.

Coffee Shop Bliss: Would you like a gluten-free muffin with that?

Corporate chain and independent coffee shops across the country in cities both large and small have at least one delicious gluten-free baked good to enjoy with a beverage. They either make their own on-site or purchase from local suppliers.

Gluten-Free Bakeries:

It will be common to find a large variety of gluten-free bakeries in most metropolitan cities to adequately serve the gluten-free population. Walking into many large supermarket bakeries to buy a fresh baked gluten-free cookie, muffin, or bread from the case is commonplace.

Marketing and Advertising:

Multi-million dollar advertising agencies have caught the wave and incorporate the gluten-free designation into the package graphic design of many leading supermarket brands that can make that claim. They not only want to be competitive in capturing the large segment of the population that is now living gluten-free, they simply want to promote many of their products as being healthy and easier to digest because they are gluten-free. Gluten-free marketing lingo has become common as it was in the early days of the "all natural" and "organic" food movements.

Schools for Children:

When a student is being registered for school, from elementary through college, it's standard operating procedure to ask if the student will require gluten-free meals so the school can develop a strategic plan for the school year to accommodate the needs more efficiently. The majority of schools have designed their meal programs in a way that is healthy and efficient in meeting the needs of the children with special diets.

Hospitals:
Hospital meal programs and cafeterias have designated gluten-free meal options and even space in the kitchen to avoid cross-contact while preparing gluten-free meals for patients and visitors.

Medications:
Drug manufacturers have reformulated most if not all of their products that previously contained gluten to be gluten-free, so there is never a question regarding gluten-free status for the patient or consumer.

Personal Hygiene Products:
Labeling practices for soaps, shampoos, cosmetics, and other topical products have adopted a set of standard voluntary guidelines for manufacturers to label their products as gluten-free. Many products have been reformulated to be gluten-free versions to accommodate a growing segment of the population that chooses to purchase hygiene products that are gluten-free.

Testing For Celiac Disease Among Children:
Screening for the celiac gene is included in a standard panel of many tests carried out on babies. When the test indicates positive, preventative measures are taken with respect to following a gluten-free diet.

Psychiatry and Psychology:
It's common practice that professionals consider intestinal health as a pivotal aspect of emotional well-being and will inquire about their patient's diet first to rule out any connection

between intestinal health and behavioral problems before prescribing medication. More patients adopt a gluten-free diet as part of the initial counseling phase when warranted or are encouraged to get tested for celiac disease or gluten-intolerance in connection with early treatment.

Awareness:

The national focus on building awareness of celiac disease and gluten-intolerance to help increase diagnosis rates among individuals has shifted to include a dominant role of early prevention of celiac disease with screening and following a gluten-free diet. Rates of osteoporosis, other bone diseases, and previous complications with gluten-intolerance and celiac disease have fallen dramatically as a result of early diagnosis and prevention.

ART & SCIENCE: GLUTEN-FREE CHEMISTRY AND SUBSTITUTION TIPS

- Before beginning a gluten-free baking recipe, what should you look for?
- What's a good trick for preventing your pie crust dough from breaking apart when rolling it out?
- Can you "overwork" gluten-free dough?
- What can help your gluten-free bread achieve a better rise?
- How can you best preserve your gluten-free bread?
- Why is foil often used in gluten-free baking?
- Is there a secret to measuring gluten-free flour?
- If your gluten-free baked recipes turn out differently each time you make them, what could be the reason?
- If you are dairy-intolerant, what can you use in place of milk in gluten-free baking?
- What should you keep in mind when cooking gluten-free grains?
- What are some tips that can save you money when eating gluten-free?

Before beginning a gluten-free baking recipe, what should you look for?

You will find that gluten-free cookbooks call for certain ingredients in the recipe, such as milk, butter, and eggs, to be at room temperature before blending them together and/or incorporating them into the recipe. Why? Because when these ingredients have lost their "chill" and are neutral in temperature, they blend together better with the rest of the recipe's ingredients and can help achieve better overall results for gluten-free baked goods. Using ingredients cold can be a hard habit to break when you are used to traditional baking, but try to get in the habit of taking your cold ingredients from the refrigerator before you start and allow them to reach room temperature before you need them. They can continue to warm up while you are working on other aspects of the recipe. By the time you are ready to incorporate them, they should be at room temperature, and should blend well with your gluten-free ingredients.

What's a good trick for preventing your pie crust dough from breaking apart when rolling it out?

Through trial and error, many gluten-free cookbooks and chefs have discovered and agree that using plastic wrap can work wonders. When you're ready to roll out your gluten-free pastry dough, place the dough ball on a sheet of plastic wrap and begin to pat it down with your hands. Then lay another sheet of plastic wrap on top and carefully roll out your dough with a rolling pin, adjusting the plastic wrap if you need to as you go. This will help keep sticky gluten-free pastry dough from sticking to the rolling pin and can help create a smoother crust.

Can you "overwork" gluten-free dough?

"Working the dough" is a common term used to describe the kneading process of traditional gluten-based yeast bread—the kneading process helps develop the gluten. However, gluten-free bread dough is not kneaded, it's mixed. Gluten-free bread dough is more aptly described as a bread batter; similar to a cake batter, but thicker and stickier. While you should follow the recipe's mixing instructions for your gluten-free bread, the suggested time to stop mixing is more of a guideline that says you are good to move on to the next step. Even though you can over-mix a batter to the point where the results would no longer be optimal, generally speaking, gluten-free baking science says you can't "overwork" the dough because there is no gluten.

What can help your gluten-free bread achieve a better rise?

It's common practice to cover a traditional gluten-loaf with a towel and seek the warmest spot in the kitchen for the dough to rise. On top of the refrigerator is often just the place. And while tops of refrigerators also serve gluten-free yeast bread batters well, gluten-free baking experts are finding ingenious ways to enhance a gluten-free rise. While there are many expert opinions on this topic, Certified Master Baker and gluten-free baking expert Richard Coppedge of the Culinary Institute of America in Hyde Park, New York, offers a unique hint. He finds that a humid environment can help achieve a better gluten-free batter rise. So, should you move to Florida? Well, you could, but try creating a moist environment in your microwave first. Coppedge recommends heating water in a microwave to produce a warm, humid environment, then placing your loaf pan inside the microwave to rise.

How can you best preserve your gluten-free bread?

You will find that fresh gluten-free baked bread is at its best right out of the oven. However, it's common to find that gluten-free bread begins to harden and loose its moisture if it remains on the counter too long. To best preserve your loaf, slice your bread all at once after it cools, place it in tightly sealed freezer bags, and freeze. Double bag if your freezer is known to impart a hint of unsavory freezer burn.

Gluten-free bread typically freezes well for long periods, and slices can be thawed and used on demand—however, you will need to toast most slices. Be careful not to wait too long to freeze your bread once it's baked; even just a few hours can be too long and the bread can pass its prime. A good rule to remember: Freeze early so you can enjoy later! Also, keep this tip in mind when bringing fresh baked gluten-free bread home from a local bakery.

Why is foil often used in gluten-free baking?

You will find that many gluten-free bread recipes call for foil to be placed over the loaf while it's baking, sometimes for as long as 40 to 50 minutes. Gluten-free breads can be prone to browning quickly, and covering with foil can help keep the loaf from over-browning.

Is there a secret to measuring gluten-free flours?

Gluten-free baking experts are quick to recommend that you pay close attention to measuring your flours and starches. No eyeballing! This means filling your measuring cup full, but no packing it down. Scrape the top of the measuring cup with a flat edged implement like a knife to remove the excess. This same guideline applies to measuring spoons.

While these are helpful strategies, keep in mind that ten people can measure a cup of flour and a food scale will reveal ten different weights. Why? Because the flour or starch can have pockets of air that may not be visible and this air is included in your measurement. This is why pastry chefs often use scales to weigh their dry ingredients to ensure accuracy. So, if you're passionate about detail and accuracy, you may want to take your measuring prowess up a notch by investing in a kitchen scale that will weigh your ingredients. This way you can be assured that you are getting a true measurement for your dry ingredients. Your gluten-free recipe will thank you for it by providing better results!

If your gluten-free baked recipes turn out differently each time you make them, what could be the reason?

This is a common complaint from many gluten-free baking beginners. Gluten-free baking is often more science than art, and while environmental factors like humidity or even altitude can have an impact on your baked goods, your measuring accuracy (or lack thereof) is most likely the culprit. Pay close attention to measuring your ingredients, both dry and wet, as accurately as you can. Also, the temperature of the ingredients could be a factor. Remember that many gluten-free recipes call for certain ingredients like milk, butter, eggs, and water to be at room temperature before incorporating them into the recipe. If you begin with cold ingredients straight from the refrigerator, you could have different results. Even ovens and their temperature calibrations can have an effect. Get to know your oven well so you can better predict how it will perform for you in making gluten-free baked goods.

If you are dairy-intolerant, what can you use in place of milk in gluten-free baking?

Gluten-free cookbooks and product manufacturers are aware that dairy-intolerance is common among gluten-intolerant individuals, and you will find that many of their recipes will offer dairy-free suggestions even though the original recipe may call for milk. It is common to find that rice milk, soy milk, almond milk, or even water can make excellent replacements, depending on the recipe.

Sometimes a recipe will call for the same amount of the nondairy alternative as it did for the dairy, which reveals that this type of substitution will not have a negative impact on the recipe—it implies that the other ingredients are more pivotal. Even coconut milk is sometimes suggested, particularly in nonbaked items such as puddings. But when you don't see a dairy-free suggestion for a recipe on a manufacturer's product recipe, call them for a suggestion or opt to experiment by replacing the milk with your own dairy-free alternative, and see what happens! Experimentation is alive and well in gluten- and dairy-free baking.

What should you keep in mind when cooking gluten-free grains?

Because cooking gluten-free grains such as amaranth, quinoa, millet, or teff are typically unfamiliar territory for the gluten-free beginner (and can be tricky even for a seasoned veteran), it can be intimidating to try these grains—but if you don't, you'll let your gluten-free cooking adventures be stopped short. When reading package instructions and following cookbook recipes using these grains, you'll soon find that they are not at all daunting and can be a joy to cook. They offer such a bounty of recipes, flavor, and nutritious versatility, don't let unfamiliarity steer you away from trying these marvelous staples. And with more use, you can uncover insightful tips from culinary experts. For example, quinoa cooks and fluffs up like rice. But Lorna Sass in her cookbook *Whole Grains Every Day Every Way* suggests also that this grain will cook best when it is boiled in an ample amount of water, like you would cook pasta. Adding these grains to your roster offers so many more opportunities for you to experiment and find gluten-free foods you love; though you're unfamiliar with cooking them, a little experimentation can wind up both fun and profitable.

What are some tips that can save you money when eating gluten-free?

For the typical person living gluten-free, food costs are all around higher and saving money with this lifestyle is both an art as well as a science, because it involves creativity and logic. So, what can you do to save money over the long run? If you like to bake and cook at home, you're already a step ahead. Pressures on the pocketbook can nudge you back into the kitchen, where you can make many gluten-free foods in advance and freeze them for later enjoyment. Consider the following:

- When making your flour blends for baking, invest in the gluten-free flours you need and create a large batch at once. Store the blends well in tightly sealed containers that are protected from sunlight. Refrigeration nearly always helps. And always similarly protect your leftover ingredients that didn't make it into the blend for future use. With a large batch of your all-purpose gluten-free flour blend at the ready, you can easily make your gluten-free baked goods whenever you want. But if a pre-made flour blend is not always available, the urge to buy pre-made, gluten-free baked goods—which are naturally more expensive— can be alluring. When you figure the arithmetic for making your own gluten-free breads, muffins, and cookies etc. based on price per serving and compare them to pre-made baked goods, you'll easily find you will save money by eating at home.
- If you purchase foods online, try to buy in bulk so you save on shipping costs.
- Organize gluten-free cooking parties using your kitchen or a friend's kitchen (particularly if you have a friend with a very large kitchen). Invite friends, family, or members of your local support group to select recipes that you can all make in big

batches and divide amongst yourselves. Each person contributes one or more ingredients into the pool and then you can all enjoy baking up a storm together, having fun, and saving money all at the same time!

- Avoid impulse purchases based on hunger pangs throughout the day by always having snacks available to tide you over until the next meal. Planning ahead for snack emergencies can save big over time.
- Always watch for sales! Even though you may not need your favorite gluten-free pasta at the time you find it on sale, buy it now in bulk because you'll use it later, and you might as well reap the price savings now rather than lose them.

GLUTEN-FREE FOOD COMPANY DIRECTORY

Listed is a sampling of companies that are specialty gluten-free companies by design or they manufacture one or more gluten-free products in addition to their regular product line. Most companies have national product distribution in the United States. Remember: If you don't find a gluten-free designation on a package or website, call the manufacturer to confirm.

United States

1-2-3 Gluten Free Inc.	412-683-2424	www.123glutenfree.com
AllerEnergy	513-478-4466	www.allerenergy.com
AlpineAire Foods	800-322-6325	www.aa-foods.com
AltiPlano Gold	415-928-9928	www.altiplangold.com
Amazing Grains Grower Cooperative	877-278-6585	wwwamazinggrains.com
Amy's Kitchen Inc.	707-578-7188	www.amyskitchen.com
Ancient Harvest Quinoa Corporation	310-217-8125	www.quinoa.com
Annie Chun's Inc.	415-479-8272	www.anniechun.com
Annie's Homegrown Inc.	800-288-1089	www.annies.com
Annie's Naturals	800-288-1089	www.anniesnaturals.com
Applegate Farms	866-587-5858	www.applegatefarms.com
Arico Natural Foods Company	503-259-0871	www.aricofoods.com
Arrowhead Mills	800-434-4246	www.arrowheadmills.com
Authentic Foods	800-806-4737	www.authenticfoods.com
Barbara's Bakery	707-765-2273	www.barbarasbakery.com

Bakery on Main	888-533-8118	www.bakeryonmain.com
Bard's Tale Beer Company LLC	816-272-2015	www.bardsbeer.com
Bête Noire Chocolates	303-399-4876	www.betenoirechocolates.com
Bionaturae	860-642-6996	www.bionaturae.com
Blue Diamond Growers	800-987-2329	www.bluediamond.com
Bob's Red Mill Natural Foods Inc.	800-553-2258	www.bobsredmill.com
BumbleBar Foods, Inc.	888-453-3369	www.bumblebar.com
Breads from Anna	877-354-3886	www.glutenevolution.com
The Cape Cod Potato Chip Co.	888-881-2447	www.capecodchips.com
Celia's Gourmet	866-938-5020	www.wheatfreefood.com
Chebe Bread	800-217-9510	www.chebe.com
Daddy Sam's	612-669-0218	www.daddysams.com
De Boles	800-434-4246	www.hain-celestial.com
The Dietary Shoppe Inc.	215-242-5302	www.dietaryshoppe.com
Dietary Specialties	888-640-2800	www.dietspec.com
Dowd & Rogers Inc.	816-451-6490	www.dowdandrogers.com
Dr. Praeger's Sensible Foods	877-772-3437	www.drpraegers.com
Eden Foods	800-248-0320	www.edenfoods.com
Edward & Sons Trading Co. Inc.	805-684-8500	www.edwardsandsons.com
Ener-G Foods	800-331-5222	www.ener-g.com
Enjoy Life Foods	888-503-6569	www.enjoylifefoods.com
Erewhon	800-422-1125	www.usmillsinc.com
Ethnic Gourmet	800-434-4246	www.ethnicgourmet.com
Food for Life Baking Company	800-797-5090	www.foodforlife.com
Foods by George LLC	201-612-9700	www.foodsbygeorge.com
Fortitude Brands LLC	866-664-5883	www.fortitudebrands.com
GardenSpot's Finest	800-829-5100	www.gardenspotsfinest.com
Gifts of Nature	888-275-0003	www.giftsofnature.net
Gillian's Foods, Inc.	781-586-0086	www.gilliansfoods.com
GlutenFreeda Foods Inc.	360-378-3675	www.glutenfreeda.com
Gluten-Free Kneads	512-706-1775	www.glutenfreekneads.com

Gluten Free Oats	307-754-2058	www.glutenfreeoats.com
Gluten-Free Pantry/Glutino USA	800-291-8386	www.glutenfreepantry.com
Gluten-Free Trading Company	888-993-9933	www.gluten-free.net
Grainaissance	800-472-4697	www.grainaissance.com
Hain Pure Foods	800-434-4246	www.hainpurefoods.com
Health Valley	800-434-4246	www.healthvalley.com
Heartland's Finest	888-658-8909	www.heartlandsfinest.com
Hodgson Mill	800-525-0177	www.hodgsonmill.com
Hol-Grain	800-551-3245	www.conradricemill.com
Ian's Natural Foods	978-989-0601	www.iansnatualfoods.com
Imagine Foods	800-434-4246	www.imaginefoods.com
Inca Organics	866-328-4622	www.incaorganics.com
Josef's Gluten-Free	718-599-0707	www.josefsglutenfree.com
Kind Fruit + Nut Bars	212-616-3006	www.kindsnacks.com
Lakefront Brewery, Inc.	414-372-8800	www.lakefrontbrewery.com
Lärabar/Humm Foods, Inc.	877-527-2227	www.larabar.com
Lotus Foods	866-972-6879	www.lotusfoods.com
Lundberg Family Farms	530-882-4551	www.lundberg.com
Manischewitz	201-333-3700	www.manischewitz.com
Mariposa Baking Company	510-868-1639	www.mariposabaking.com
Marlene's Mixes	903-839-3892	www.marlenesmixes.com
Mary's Gone Crackers	888-258-1250	www.marysgonecrackers.com
Masuya (USA) Inc.	916-979-7872	www.masuyanaturally.com
Mimi's Gourmet	201-399-4302	www.mimisgourmet.com
Miss Roben's	800-891-0083	www.allergygrocer.com
Mona's Gluten-Free	866-486-0701	www.madebymona.com
Mr. Ritt's Bakery	877-677-4887	www.mrritts.com
Mr. Spice	800-728-2348	www.mrspice.com
Namaste Foods	866-258-9493	www.namastefoods.com
Nana's Cookie Company	800-836-7534	www.healthycrowd.com
Nature's Hilights Inc.	800-313-6454	www.natures-hilights.com

Natures Path Foods Inc.	888-808-9505	www.naturespath.com
Nu-World Amaranth	877-692-8899	www.nuworldfamily.com
Organic Food Bar	888-808-8276	www.organicfoodbar.com
Oskri Organics	800-628-1110	www.oskri.com
Pacific Foods	503-692-9666	www.pacificfoods.com
Pamela's Products	707-462-6605	www.pamelasproducts.com
Papadini/Adrienne's Gourmet Foods	805-964-6848	www.adriennes.com
Pear Bars	509-427-4433	www.gorgedelights.com
Perky's Natural Foods	888-473-7597	www.perkysnaturalfoods.com
Pinnacle Gold	707-509-4528	www.celiac.com
Pure Bar	888-568-PURE	www.thepurebar.com
Ramapo Valley Brewer	866-932-5918	www.ramapovalleybrewery.com
San-J International	800-446-5500	www.san-j.com
Simply Coconut	719-596-4875	www.simplycoconut.com
Spring Bakehouse	866-938-5020	www.wheatfreefood.com
Sunstart Bakery	630-851-2111	www.sunstartbakery.com
Sylvan Border Farm	800-297-5399	www.sylvanborderfarm.com
Tandoor Chef	905-694-9550	www.deepfoods.com
The Birkett Mills	315-536-3311	www.thebirkettmills.com
The Republic of Tea	800-298-4832	www.republicoftea.com
The Ruby Range	970-577-0888	www.therubyrange.com
The Teff Company	888-822-2221	www.teffco.com
Thai Kitchen	800-967-7424	www.thaikitchen.com
Tom Sawyer Gluten-Free Products	877-372-8800	www.glutenfreeflour.com
Van's International	323-585-5581	www.vanswaffles.com
Whole Foods Market Inc.	512-477-4455	www.wholefoodsmarket.com
White Mountain Farm	800-364-3019	www.whitemountainfarm.com

Canada

Cheecha Krackles	877-243-3242	www.cheech.ca
Château Cream Hill Estates Ltd.	866-727-3628	www.creamhillestates.com
Cream of the Crop	877-259-7491	www.alimentstrigone.com
El Peto Products Ltd.	800-387-4064	www.elpeto.com
FarmPure Foods	306-791-3770	www.farmpure.com
Kingsmill Foods	905-888-5836	www.canbrands.ca
Kinnikinnick Foods	877-503-4466	www.kinnikinnick.com
La Messagere	800-789-5962	www.baluchon.com/bnf
LifeSoy	905-831-5433	www.lifemax.com
Lifestream Natural Foods	888-808-9505	www.naturespath.com
Lorenzo's Specialty Foods Ltd.	866-639-1711	www.lorenzosfoods.ca
Micah's Favourite	905-898-0739	www.micahsfavourite.com
Natural Food Mill Bakery	800-353-3178	www.naturalfoodmill.com
Nature's Path/EnviorKidz	888-808-9505	www.naturespath.com
Northern Quinoa Corporation	866-368-9304	www.quinoa.com
Pastariso	905-451-7423	www.maplegrovefoods.com
Tinkyada Pasta Joy	416-609-0016	www.tinkyada.com

Other Countries

Barkat/Glutano (United Kingdom)	020 8953 4444	www.glutenfreefoods.co.uk
Glutafin (United Kingdom)	0845 603 9895	www.glutafin.co.uk
Leda Nutrition (Australia)	617 5530 4808	www.ledanutrition.com
Orgran (Australia)	03 9776 9044	www.orgran.com
Real Foods (Australia)	61 2 8595 6600	www.cornthins.com

Bibliography

Barrett, Amanda, "Introducing Gluten to an Infant's Diet Too Soon— or Too Late—May Raise the Risk of Celiac Disease in Predisposed Children," New York University Medical Center, 2006.

Case, Shelley, *Gluten-Free Diet—A Comprehensive Resource Guide*, Saskatchewan, Case Nutrition Consulting, 2006.

Crowe, Jeanne Patricia, *Help Yourself to Gluten Free Medication*, article found at http://www.alamoceliac.org/actipspoison.html, April 16, 2007.

Dyuff, Roberta Larson, *American Dietic Association Complete Food and Nutrition Guide, Revised & Updated 3rd Edition*, John Wiley and Sons, Inc. 2006.

Fenster, Carol, *Gluten-Free 101: Easy, Basic Dishes Without Wheat*, Savory Palate, Inc., 2006.

Green, Peter H.R., *Celiac Disease: A Hidden Epidemic*, New York: HarperCollins Publishers, 2006.

Herbst, Sharon Tyler, *The New Food Lover's Companion*, 3rd Addition, New York: Barron's Educational Series, 2001.

Laginess, Anne and summarized by Tom & Carolyn Sullivan, *Finding Gluten-Free Pharmaceuticals*, Michigan, Tri-County Celiac Sprue Support Group, April/May 2000.

MayoClinic.com, *Celiac Disease*, Mayo Foundation for Medical Education and Research, 2006.

MedicalNewsToday.com, *No Link Found Between Autism and Celiac Disease*, May 5, 2007.

Phillips, Kyle, *Your Guide to Italian Cuisine: The Pasta Shapes*

Gallery, About.com, 2007.

Sass, Lorna, *Whole Grains Every Day Every Way*, New York: Clarkson Potter, 2006.

Science Daily, *Mayo Clinic Discovers Potential Link Between Celiac Disease and Cognitive Decline*, Mayo Clinic, October 12, 2006.

Index

C

whipped cream, 88
whiskey, 67
white bean flour, 222
white flour, 76
White Mountain Farm, 107
  contact information, 320
white rice, 287
white rice flour, 76, 130, 221
white vs. brown flours and
  starches, 43
Whole Foods Market, 111, 119,
  136, 141
  contact information, 320
*Whole Grains Everyday Every
  Way* (Sass), 126, 235, 314
wine, 68
Wizard's, 117
work, gluten-free diet and
  boss and coworkers, 265—266
  business meetings, 267–268
  cross-contact and, 266–267
  snacks, 268–269
Wrigley's gum, 71

X
xantham gum, 31, 132–133,
  140, 230–231
Xylotol, 287

Y
yeast allergies, 273
yimi, 125

yogurt, 88
Yosemite National Park, 204
yucca, 132

About the Author

Suzanne Bowland has been living gluten-free for more than six years since she discovered her gluten-intolerance in 2001. A food and hospitality industry veteran, Bowland is founder and president of GF Culinary Productions, Inc., a company devoted to building awareness of the gluten-free lifestyle nationwide from the perspective of abundant options, great taste, and sound nutrition. Bowland produces gluten-free culinary education special events for the public featuring gluten-free baking and cooking classes conducted by notable culinary institute chef-instructors, restaurant chefs, cookbook authors, and industry experts. The Gluten-Free Culinary Summit and the Art & Science of Gluten-Free Gastronomy Lecture Series are two of many events produced by Bowland. Her website is www.theglutenfreelifestyle.com. She lives in Colorado.